A Song in the Night

www.nanatalese.com

DOUBLEDAY is a registered trademark of Random House, Inc.
Nan A. Talese and the colophon are trademarks of
Random House, Inc.

Book design by Pei Loi Koay
Jacket design by Emily Mahon

Library of Congress Cataloging-in-Publication Data
Massie, Robert, 1956–
A song in the night : a memoir of resilience / Bob Massie. —
1st U.S. ed.
p. cm.
1. Massie, Robert, 1956—Health. 2. HIV-positive
persons—United States—Biography. 3. Hemophiliacs—
United States—Biography. 4. Blood—Transfusion—
Complications—United States. I. Title.
RC606.55.M37A3 2012
362.19697'920092—dc23
[B]
2012004971

ISBN 978-0-385-53575-5

MANUFACTURED IN THE UNITED STATES OF AMERICA

3 5 7 9 10 8 6 4 2

First Edition

This book is dedicated

*

to Anne,

my love, my life

*

and to Kate,

my gift, my joy

Did things just happen, or did we make things come about? I knew that nothing we were living through had just come to pass. We had willed it all, worked for it, never given up, never let go of the basic ideas. Yes, we had believed—belief had been fundamental—but we had backed it up with endless hard work, and learned how to do things together, and to accommodate the fears and interests of others, and to survive the sarcasm and disbelief of those who regarded themselves as more knowledgeable than ourselves about what they called the real world, and we just kept on going on and on until at last the impossible became first feasible, then real, and finally inevitable.

ALBIE SACHS,

JUSTICE OF THE SOUTH AFRICAN

CONSTITUTIONAL COURT

Contents

A Song in the Night

CHAPTER ONE

Love AND *Pain*

From my earliest moments, my life was marked by deep joy interrupted regularly by searing physical pain. A strange pairing, perhaps, but not wholly uncommon. The pleasures of my childhood were frequent and pure. I had a natural tendency toward exuberance; I often experienced unadorned delight at the most normal of moments. I felt the deep devotion of others, beginning with my parents, who made me feel safe even when I was in misery.

I was born with a severe genetic illness, classical hemophilia, in which the absence or malfunction of a single protein known as Factor VIII interrupts the process of coagulation that stops bleeding. As a result, blood that might normally clot in five minutes instead takes forty-five minutes to an hour or even longer. Of course this causes problems with cuts and bruising, both of which take longer than usual to heal. The most dangerous problem, of which most people are unaware, is internal joint bleeding. This problem causes severe, extremely painful swelling of the joints, which in my case gradually destroyed my knees and ankles. For this reason I have almost no memories of what it was like to be able to skip or to run around my house or my backyard—except for one particular incident.

In the early 1960s we were living in a small house on Northampton Drive in White Plains, New York. We had a swing and a sandbox in the backyard and a weeping willow next to the garage. I conducted experiments at the breakfast table, such as pouring my chocolate milk into my orange juice on the theory that if they tasted good separately, they would taste even better in combination. I put cloth napkins over the lamps in the living room to see what would happen, and realized when they started to turn brown and emit wisps of smoke that this was probably not a good idea.

When I was four—about the time John F. Kennedy became president—my parents enrolled me in a tiny nursery school set up in an old home tucked away from the street. A large area of grass and trees encircled the home, and on one corner of the property sat a small menagerie of farm animals in various pens and cages. Once a week we would visit these animals, which included an old horse, a few indifferent rabbits, and a small, grumpy goat.

Daily recess, held on the yard directly in front of the old home, brought its own pleasures and challenges. In the middle of the once elegant grass sat an old-fashioned red fire truck sunk past its axles in the dirt. It had been donated to the school as a climbing structure. Stripped of its tools and hoses and left open to the elements, the fire truck had tarnished brass fixtures and cracked leather seats. Still, this wreck appeared to our eyes as the most magnificent chariot on earth. Everyone wanted to sit in the driver's seat. The honor fell each day to the fastest runner.

We would line up on the porch of the old house, jostling like young thoroughbreds at a starting gate, forbidden to move until the signal was given. Released, we would bound down the steps and race over the grass toward the fire truck, laughing and gulping for air. I lost that sprint many times, but on one glorious day I made it to the truck first.

I can still recall the blessed sensation of what it is like to run: the intoxication of blurred grass beneath my feet, the exhilaration of momentary flight as the back foot leaves the ground just before the front one touches down, the overall thrill as one's vision is smudged by speed.

When I vaulted into the driver's seat, I seized the great steering wheel with both hands and would not yield my place until recess had ended. As I trudged slowly back to the school, I let my classmates dash ahead.

Entering the front door of the school, I turned to look one more time at the fire truck on the lawn. The sunlight made the red paint on the truck glow like fire. Why is that image burned in my memory? Perhaps it was a premonition that I was saying goodbye to a form of pleasure that would never be mine again.

*

In the months following, the joint bleedings got much worse. Capillaries inside a muscle or a joint would break and pressure would build inside a knee or an ankle until I became delirious with pain. Recovery took weeks. Within a year of nursery school, the bleedings had become so frequent and so brutal that I lost the ability to walk.

In the fall of 1962, when I was six, my biggest choice was who to be at Halloween. I had spent hours watching Roy Rogers, the most famous cowboy on television, dashing around on his horse, Trigger, shooting the guns out of the hands of villains (but never injuring them). I also was captivated by the space program. In the end I decided that the best choice would be the hero who stood for "Truth, Justice, and the American Way": Superman.

This meant that I would need a store-bought costume. My mother didn't like such things, but she complied and brought one home. I thought it looked glorious: a shirt and leggings in blue, shorts and flowing cape in red, and a shiny yellow belt. I was so taken with it—especially the huge "*S*" emblazoned across my chest—that my mother felt it necessary to read, and reread, the printed warning that the costume *did* not and *could* not under *any* circumstances confer special powers such as flying.

I didn't have any illusions about that; I just wanted to walk around in it and collect candy and admiration. By that time I had been in a full-length leg brace for a year, moving stiffly across the floor; soon both legs would be locked. Most children reacted with fear when they met me, and I had to wrestle with the sting of their rejection. This Halloween, however, I decided I would not care. They would not see a boy in a brace but the Man of Steel.

The night before, however, my left knee swelled suddenly and violently, so I was trapped in terrible pain on the couch in our living room. On Halloween, I stubbornly put the costume on anyway. Maybe it would bestow a few powers to carry me through the evening.

My father, reading the dejection on my face, offered to push me in my wheelchair from house to house, or even carry me. I declined. Superman in a wheelchair just didn't make sense. I stayed on the couch, trying to appear nonchalant. Local children came to the door, and my mother brought a few of them in so that they could admire my costume. They were so clearly shocked and embarrassed that I quickly forbade her to admit anyone else.

The only remaining admirer was my uncle Kim, who came for dinner. My parents intercepted him in the front yard, and when he walked in he made a huge display of how impressed he was to meet Superman in person. He asked me about my adventures and wanted to know why I had chosen to pay a visit to, of all people, his useless brother.

When I removed the costume later that evening, I shouted as I tried to slide it past my hot and throbbing knee. That night, unable to sleep because of my suffering, I sat by myself in my bedroom, staring out the dark window above my bed. The whole evening had been a disaster. There was no way to relive it or to retrieve it. It was gone forever. It took a long time for my breathing and my heartache to settle.

Slowly the days passed, and new happiness approached. With the arrival of Thanksgiving and Christmas, I gradually put the Halloween incident behind me. Tomorrow, I told myself, would be different. There were still things to look forward to. And I knew, somehow, that the future would contain many surprises. I carefully protected my unspoken dreams, each too fragile to be mentioned. Some of them seemed so unlikely that I did not want to be ridiculed for entertaining them. And the deepest hope, held like a jewel in my heart of hearts, was that maybe, *maybe,* somehow, someday, I would again step free of those leg braces—and walk.

*

Though hemophilia is a hereditary illness, it often appears without warning because of hidden genetic mutations. There had been no history of it in my family. My parents had met in 1950 in Paris, while they were both on academic scholarships. After a passionate romance that seemed destined for marriage, my father reversed course and enlisted as a lieutenant in the U.S. Navy. After three years of floating around on an aircraft carrier, he reconsidered his decision. When he returned on leave to the United States, he courted and won my mother. At the time she was living in New York, working as a researcher for *Life* magazine. Married in late 1954, they spent the last months of his service at the naval base in Jacksonville, Florida.

In early 1956 my parents discovered that they were going to have a child. My father, at the age of twenty-seven, despite multiple degrees, a Rhodes Scholarship, and a strong record as a military officer, was having a terrible time finding a job. After more than fifty interviews, he finally landed a position as a bank teller. At the last moment, he was invited to become the assistant to a distinguished journalist and author, a move that set him on the path to writing.

My parents found a tiny apartment they could afford in Eastchester, New York, and my mother spent the spring trying to get the place set up for an infant. By August the city was roiling with heat and the country's Democrats were meeting in Manhattan to nominate their presidential candidate. As someone who has cared about politics for most of his life—and who has seen many ups and downs in the electoral process—I have always found it amusing that on the day of my birth, *U.S. News & World Report* predicted that by nominating Adlai Stevenson for the second time, the Democrats would be able to overcome the popularity of the incumbent president, Dwight Eisenhower. I came into the world at noon on August 17, 1956, at New York Hospital, which overlooks the East River, in the same town and at the very moment that the Democrats were carefully planning their unintentional path to defeat.

During the first months of my life, there were subtle signs that my parents were about to face difficulties far more complex than raising a child. The use of forceps at my birth had left a large bruise, or hematoma, at the back of my neck, which took a long time to go down. My father managed to get himself reassigned to the editorial staff of *Collier's* magazine. Things seemed to be looking up—until one Sunday, the week before Christmas, the magazine's employees received telegrams saying that *Collier's* had collapsed. They had all been officially out of work since the previous Friday.

Without severance pay, insurance, or savings, my parents

were financially desperate. To buy food and pay the rent, they went on welfare, which at that time was $36 a week. My father plunged into looking for new work. Happily, he found a job in a month, this time writing book reviews for *Newsweek*.

In early January my uncle Kim came to visit, and he rolled me around my playpen and tossed me in the air while I laughed and gurgled happily. Not long after his visit I had a small bruise on my left forearm. At my next routine doctor's visit, my mother pointed out the bruise to my pediatrician, who wondered what might have caused it. He ordered a blood count, then sent us to New York Hospital for more extensive testing.

My mother, joined eventually by my father and my Swiss grandmother, waited all day and evening in the outer offices of New York's most prominent hematologist to learn the results of the tests. The doctor never came. We went back and waited all the next day. Finally, on the second evening, the doctor appeared, impeccably dressed and greatly rushed. His eyes never left the floor as he spoke to my parents. "The child has classical hemophilia," he announced, and then added enigmatically, "There will be compensations, you may be sure." With those mystifying words, he turned and left.

"I don't know what we did then," my mother wrote years later. "I can't remember leaving the hospital or finding the car in the parking lot. Somehow, we reached the safe haven of our tiny apartment with its packing crate for a table and its single kitchen chair. In one cataclysmic moment our world had been shattered. We only numbly recognized our familiar surroundings. We wept there, the three of us—Bob, my mother, and I—clinging to each other, helpless and alone. Without warning, as surely as if we had been abandoned on the bleak surface of the moon, our lives had changed. We had no idea what lay ahead."

*

Years later I learned how hard they worked over the coming months—to identify the right questions, the right doctors, the right treatments. Most of what they learned was grim. Human joints are marvels of engineering, and to supply all the muscles and tissues with oxygen and other nutrients requires an almost infinitely complex network of tiny, fragile blood vessels. No carpenter strikes a blow, no basketball player lands after a jump shot, without sending a jolt through his or her joints. Frequently these shocks cause the tiny blood vessels to break, and blood begins to leak into the cavity of the ankle, the elbow, the knee. Most human beings never feel these injuries because the coagulation system quickly plugs the leaks. As a child I used to imagine all the parts of the coagulation system speeding toward the wounded area the same way that firefighters and EMTs rush to an accident. For a child with hemophilia, however, the coagulation system breaks down. The ambulances and fire trucks all have flat tires; no one shows up at the crash site. As a result, blood slowly fills the joint cavity around the ends of bone and between strands of muscle tissue. As the amount of blood increases, the pressure builds, and the pressure brings pain, first distant and diffuse, then sharper and more focused. Eventually, when there is no more room, the joint becomes rigid, but even then the blood continues to leak; the pressure mounts, and the pain relentlessly mounts with it. When I was a child—and still, fifty years later—there were really only two things that would stop this internal bleeding: injecting Factor VIII, which enables clotting to occur, or elevating the joint and bathing it in ice, which somewhat slows the rate of bleeding.

My parents, both journalists, directed all of their love and all of their professional skills into protecting me. To become the best possible care providers for me, they felt that they needed to know everything—the medical and biochemical details of the disease, the names and advice of the best doctors, the recommended forms of care both inside and outside the hospital. They made phone calls and interviewed doctors and researchers whose names floated like the names of distant saints through the backgrounds of our conversation. My mother steeled herself against the shocked and disapproving glares she met at the grocery store, where other suburban moms looked at my bruises and concluded that she had been beating me.

Nonetheless, they surrounded me with optimism. They talked to me and played games with me and cooked my favorite foods. When my sister, Susanna, was born a few months before my second birthday, they folded her into what seemed—to me—to be our truly happy family.

It was then that we moved into our two-bedroom ranch house in White Plains, New York. For many years, whenever

I was asked about my childhood, I could mostly call up happy circumstances of my early life. It took years for me to make sense of the strange life I actually lived, a life that careened between love and pain. I could be experiencing all the normal daily pleasures of being a child when suddenly, without warning, a terrifying crisis would begin. My parents exhibited extraordinary devotion, vigilance, and discipline. Even in the most agonizing assaults, they became the vehicles through which love emerged to offer comfort, to begin the healing, and to signal that ahead there still lay hope.

Some of the incidents, I now see, were so frightening and overwhelming that my mind quickly deleted them from my active memory. When I draw them up now, decades later, I feel great grief and sorrow for the tiny boy who was subjected to such awful duress but could not yet understand why this was happening to him, and for his parents, who were powerless to protect him.

*

I only began to understand and to retain my experiences as I gained the capacity for language. I still remember the wedge of light from the hallway lighting up the warm golden ash of the slats of my crib as my parents closed the door and wished me goodnight. I recall whispering in the dark to Teddy, my twelve-inch stuffed bear, who went with me everywhere, even on those terrible nights when my parents realized that I had to be lifted from bed, bundled tenderly into the car, and driven at high speed to the hospital.

I would lie in the backseat, streetlights streaking rhythmically by overhead, and for a moment I would imagine that I was a grown-up, off to some important nighttime adventure. We would pull up to the hospital—Cross County Medical Center, in the middle of a shopping mall, just off the highway that led into Manhattan. On arrival, my parents would fill out pages of paperwork while the hematologist was called; all the time we waited, the swelling and the pain in my joint rose steadily. When he came, he would examine me and confirm my need for plasma. Only then would fresh frozen plasma—the only source of Factor VIII—be ordered from the blood bank, slowly procured, slowly thawed: more delays, more swelling.

When the plasma finally arrived and the doctor threaded the needle into a vein in my arm, a small stream of crimson blood would slide back up the tubing, indicating that the connection had been made, and the precious drops of yellow plasma would start dripping into my bloodstream, into the big veins and arteries and down through ever-smaller tributaries, taking Factor VIII within seconds to the damaged spot. This enabled healing to begin and, within hours, brought a slow end to the fire of pain.

While I sat in the small room with the white tiles, the plasma lazily dripping from its container suspended on an infusion pole, my mother sat beside me, stroking my hair, and my father stood nearby, gazing at me with sorrow, coming over from time to time to squeeze my hand. My mother kept up a stream of whispered words: *Here, look at this book, Bobby, remember this book*, she would say, trying to distract and amuse me.

My eyes focused on the golden liquid inside the tubing: drip, drip, drip.

Bobby, she said, *look at this. You will feel better. This is not going to last forever.*

Sometimes she held my face and made me look into her eyes.

And when you feel better, she said, *we will go dancing in Paris. Do you promise me that, Bobby?*

I nodded with exhaustion, though my mind was starting to picture it.

I've been there. There are lights all up and down the streets and in the restaurants, and everywhere we will find the most wonderful music and food.

I could see it. I tried to smile.

I know this will happen, Bobby, she whispered to me. *You will get big and we will go dancing in Paris. You will be big and strong and you will be able to go. Will you do that with me?*

Yes, Mommy, I said earnestly, *I will.*

It breaks my heart to think how seriously I spoke those words as a three-year-old. But I believed that someday it all would happen, and that belief carried me through my misery and terror.

The healing often took weeks to complete. When the active bleeding stopped, the body's immune and enzymatic systems would attack the blood cells that had escaped into the joint, break them down, and reabsorb them.

In theory, that should have been the end of the story. Unfortunately, each bleeding left a legacy that made another one more likely. The period of disuse caused the muscles of the joint to atrophy, so as I tried to move again, I found myself weaker, and thus more likely to apply too much stress to the newly healed joint. The enzymes that helped reabsorb the loose cells also corroded the inner lining of the joint, degrading the joint's ability to bend smoothly. Repeated bleedings and reabsorptions steadily reduced the range of motion of each affected joint. The knees and elbows particularly refused to straighten or bend all the way. So when I began to use my body again, with its slightly weaker muscles, slightly rougher and less functional joints, it was only a matter of time before another bleeding knocked me down and carried me further toward permanent damage. Without any medications to prevent these bleedings, the spiral was inevitable.

For these reasons, and because of the danger of concussion, the life expectancy of a hemophiliac when I was born was less than thirty years. Doctors grimly told my parents that the best hope was to limit my bleeding until I had completed puberty, when the end to my growth might enable my joints to stabilize.

As every season passed and I became bigger and heavier and more active, the stress on my joints increased. The number of joint bleedings and the plasma infusions to treat them steadily rose. I could see the increasing time it took to recover from each episode, and I could tell that my abilities were gradually shrinking.

My mother tried to get me to exercise. During the weeks I was in bed, she strapped me into leg-stretching contraptions prescribed by my doctors to help with my recovery. Some were quite ingenious—attached by small vises to the footboard of the bed, they had little girders that rose above the bed and ended in small pulleys. My mother would lace a small cloth boot to my ankle and connect it to a piece of rope that ran up and over the various pulleys until it reached a place where she could attach small bags of sand to the end. The treatment called for gradually increasing the weight in the sandbags so that the mild, steady pressure would gradually straighten out my crooked and locked joints.

I hated these machines. The pulleys and sandbags caused sharp discomfort. The endlessly repeated isometric exercises— just tightening and loosening my trembling muscles—never seemed to make any difference. I wore the boots as little as possible. After patiently coaxing me to use them, only to watch me kick them off, my parents would sometimes throw up their hands in frustration. "We just don't know what to do, Bobby! You *have* to use this. If you don't, your legs will bend up a little more after every bleeding. And they are *your* legs!"

Most of the time the swelling eventually went down and I could get the leg straight enough to put weight on it. And then I would forget about the incident and try to return as swiftly as possible to the pressing duties of being an energetic boy. Finally, on one occasion that I have blocked from my memory, I had such a massive bleeding that the knee slowly jackknifed. I would not be able to put weight on it again for more than seven years.

*

With a marvelous combination of sympathy and challenge, my parents helped me fight off the occasional bouts of depression that would seize me when I was confined to my bed. They brought me books and games, helped me learn to cook, and refused to let me belittle or pity myself. During the long, boring stretches of convalescence, my mother in particular constantly looked for ways to make little, demonstrable improvements. Instinctively she knew ways to cheer me up: by straightening up the pillows to support my swollen knee, by organizing my colored pencils and paper so they would be readily accessible, or by bringing me a surprise pizza. During those interminable nights when pain banished sleep, she spent hours holding my hand and telling me stories of faraway places.

My father, consumed by work, also tried heroically to reinforce my confidence and hope. He surprised me completely one day when I was about five. He came and sat on my bed, looked at my legs, which were tied up in the infernal joint-stretching pulley machine, and said to me, "I know this must be terribly hard for you, Bobby. I just wish I could cut off and give you both of my own legs."

"What?" I said, shocked.

"Well, this is the way I think about it. I have had my legs for a while now—about thirty years. I have gotten pretty good use out of them. I think it would only be fair for me to be able to exchange them for yours so that you could get around on them now."

"But why would you do that?" I asked, staring at him. I simply could not imagine that someone would be willing to make such a sacrifice.

"Well," he said, "there's really only one reason, and that's because I love you." Then he touched my head and left the room.

*

In the prison of pain, love offers the only solace. I had no words to describe what I was experiencing, no way to understand how my life compared to anyone else's. As for every child, the boundaries of my life were foreshortened to what I could see around me, how people reacted to me, what lay before me in the moment. I had no way to care for myself, to predict what was likely to happen to me, or to respond when a crisis hit. All I could do was cling to the hope that the adults around me would help me. My parents, no matter how tired and worried they must often have been, guarded me from the abyss of danger and fear that threatened almost daily to pull me in.

One particular incident illustrated their courage and tenacity in defending me. I remember standing near the side of a brightly lit classroom in elementary school filled with small desks and bulletin boards and children's drawings. For some reason a child reached forward, planted his hand in the center of my chest, and shoved me backward. I fell hard against a closed door and felt the doorknob strike me near the center of my back. Though I had the wind knocked out of me, I recovered quickly.

At the end of the day I joined my family for a drive from Westchester County to Northampton in western Massachusetts. My mother's youngest sister, Jeannine, had invited my father to give a talk at Smith College, where she was an undergraduate, and we were all excited to visit her. When we arrived at the hotel, my parents put my sister and me to sleep in a big bed.

In a few hours, however, I awoke in terrible pain. The bruise from the doorknob had swelled to the size of a goose egg, and it was rapidly getting bigger. My parents put a bag of ice on it, but they could see that the bruise was spreading across my back and under the ribs. Soon we found ourselves at Northampton's Cooley Dickinson Hospital, where my parents consulted with the doctors in the emergency room. After examining me, they all agreed that I needed an infusion of fresh frozen plasma. There was one catch: the hospital did not have any. It was the middle of the night. Both Boston and New York were many hours away.

The adults conferred quietly while I drifted into the haze of pain. I floated into a stupor, trying to hold back the panic that made me want to throw up.

When I opened my eyes later, I could not believe what I saw. My father was lying on a table in the same room, near the opposite wall. A large needle had been inserted into his arm, and his dark venous blood was draining into a sterile plastic infusion bag hung below the table. My mother came over to explain to me what was happening.

"We could not find any plasma anywhere in the hospital," she said, "and the doctors could think of only one way to get Factor VIII into you. They are going to give you whole blood."

"Whole blood?" I knew so little, but I understood that this

meant dark red blood, full of red and white cells, with only a tiny amount of Factor VIII floating around.

"Whole blood from Daddy," she explained patiently. "As soon as they have drawn enough blood from his arm, they will begin to put it into you."

I lay there and looked across the room. A few feet away, illuminated by the pale yellow light of dawn coursing through the window, lay my father, staring resolutely at the ceiling. His maroon-colored blood was flowing through a clear tube out of his arm, filling a plastic bag, destined for me. I gazed at him, and my child's mind was overwhelmed with exhaustion, and fear, and the shock of being loved so much.

My father turned his head and looked over toward me; his face was drawn with exhaustion, but he looked carefully into my eyes.

"It's going to be all right, Bobby," he said quietly. "I promise you, it's going to be all right."

CHAPTER TWO

Sound AND *Sight*

L anguage is one of the greatest human mysteries. We often forget this, because our days and our minds are so flooded with talk. Yet the search to find the right word for our experiences is constant. Anyone who has witnessed the struggle of a foreign visitor, or a small child, or a person overcome by brain damage, to find just the right word knows how hard it is to do and how rewarding to succeed.

Speech also creates telepathy. Think about it for a moment: the eyes record an object or the ears register a sound, and these are translated instantly into meaning that is not only understandable to the self but can be communicated to others. Not all sights and sounds fit into language, but when we see something and assign it a word, or when we hear a word and assign it an image, we are creating meaning—often unconsciously—in a way that shapes our emotions, our decisions, and our future. This mystery also has a darker side. If something does *not* have a name, if we, as humans, lack a way of talking about it, then the person or the object or the idea becomes largely invisible.

As children we swim in an ocean of received wisdom. We use the words we are given; we think about things in the way we are taught. The liberation of the human mind comes with the expansion of sight and sound into new and unexplored areas. By transforming sight into sound—and back again—and by introducing the raw power of our imaginations, it becomes possible to see what never was, and to imagine what has never been.

In my first years, I was primarily the recipient of experiences—of love and of pain, of joy and of suffering—for which I had little understanding and no words. As I grew I started to look past the horizon in more ways than one. My imagination steadily took hold and allowed me to connect with people and ideas that far exceeded my own limited experience.

This capacity increased through such simple experiences as a walk in the forest. Every summer my family returned to a marvelous piece of land in Maine purchased by my maternal grandparents in the early 1940s. Situated on the tip of the island of Sunshine, near Deer Isle, it became our refuge from the world, the forest hideaway where we lived in harmony with the daily rhythms of tide and wind, rain and sun. Our tiny log cabin was near a beach, where all the local children, including my newest sister, Elizabeth, went to swim in the bone-chilling seawater.

Part of the joy of this place was that everyone could hike back and forth, through the woods and along the beach, to explore the nature around them. Everyone, that is, but me. To make up for my difficulties, my parents and friends sometimes tried to organize a special expedition to the point at the very end of the property, from which one could see all the islands in the area at once.

These rare expeditions were fraught with the danger of falling, of twisting an ankle or striking a joint on stone. The trail ran down a lengthy forest path lined with pine needles, then along an ancient moss-padded logging road, before emerging abruptly onto the hot white sand of a small beach. From there we would edge along the lapping water toward the east, up and over ledges, across patches of sand and shells and dried-out rockweed, and sometimes right through the salt flats decorated with pale green and lavender sea heather.

My father would load me into a wheelbarrow for the first stage of the expedition. He steered me carefully around the exposed roots so as not to risk tossing me out. When we reached the beach, he carried me. I remember the reassuringly familiar discomfort of his prickly wool sweater, the strength of his arms and shoulders (holding me firmly, with power to spare), and the smell of his tanned neck and unshaven cheek as he guided his feet, step by step, to the firmest spot.

When we came close to the point, he would let me try to walk, though my two full-length leg braces made this difficult. The braces had been painstakingly constructed by a specialist, who had molded and shaped the intricate steel and aluminum and leather parts to fit each leg so that I could move upright, though only slowly and with difficulty. Every morning I strapped them on, tightening the straps and buckles over my shins and thighs and knees, tying the laces of the brown oxford shoes into which the ends of the braces were bolted, straightening the knee joints out, and sliding the ingenious square locking devices down and over the joints so my legs would not buckle. I then pulled up the pants that had been carefully widened and adapted by my mother.

If I stood still, the machinery of my locomotion remained hidden; only when I started to move was the secret revealed. I would swing each limb forward, one after the other, tracing a slight sideways arc to the left, then to the right, then to the left again. In the summer I sometimes felt comfortable enough with my friends and family to wear shorts, thus fully exposing my atrophied and mechanical legs. For most people it was too shocking, and I did not want others to be uncomfortable—or to reject me.

I struggled to walk over rocks and sand and seaweed. My sisters and friends, fleet-footed and full of words of encouragement, would hop ahead of me, cheering each small advance. With canes, walking sticks, and the sturdy hands of both parents, I finally made it, and then I took in the sights and smells, the glittering waters and cleansing wind.

Behind me were the lichen-encrusted pines, firs, and spruces and the sun-splashed clearings of long grass and wildflowers. Below me lay an array of huge boulders, remnants of a molten primeval stew now cooled into granite dappled black and gray, white and pink. These immense boulders had been cracked and buffed by a thousand centuries of glaciers and storms and tides. The sea continued its work even in our presence. The water would strike sharply in slaps and pops and then withdraw with a scouring hiss through the crevices of each protruding stone.

When I finally reached my destination, on a strip of sand and stone that advanced far into the channel, I could see everything. To my right rose the dark and brooding peak of Isle au Haut surrounded by the restless waters of Penobscot Bay. Rank upon rank of waves and swells, tufted with white, swept by swiftly and rhythmically. To my left stretched the blue-black expanse of Jericho Bay, speckled with the spray-painted hues of thousands of lobster buoys. At the water's distant edge rose the majestic hills and mountains of midcoast Maine—Blue Hill, Mount Desert, and all of their lesser attendants.

Straight ahead I could see the two mysterious landmasses of Marshall and Swan's Islands. I could hear the tall red bell buoy anchored miles ahead of me ringing like a Zen sea chime. On some days the islands were hidden by fog, and on others they were so clearly spotlighted by sunlight that I could almost count the trees lining the shore.

Between the two islands, I could just make out the steady line separating pale blue sky from the gray-green of the water. It was this horizon that attracted my eyes and excited my dreams about the future. I pictured myself in a sharp wooden sailboat, slicing through the waves, streaking past the islands until I reached the ultimate freedom of open ocean and all the unknowable beauty that lay beyond. That moment might seem impossible from where I was standing, but I willfully and joyfully pictured it anyway. What I could see with my eyes blurred with what I could see in my mind.

In a sense, I was being introduced to the elementary building block of faith and hope, the belief that what I hoped for but could not see would come to pass. I may be here, I told myself, temporarily confined by my braces and by the present, but someday I will be there, moving with grace through a whole new future.

*

There were other horizons I hoped to cross, including the horizon of time. I grew up in the generation after World War II when Americans instinctively believed that every problem would eventually yield to technology. To a child bound to crutches, leg braces, and wheelchairs, science offered the thrilling hope of eventual release. I was unfamiliar with the troubling moral complexities of technologies such as the atomic bomb; for me the domain of science was idealistic and optimistic to its core. If machines could do the work of a thousand men, if new chemicals and drugs could alter nature and combat disease, then surely it was only a matter of time before someone announced a cure for hemophilia.

My interest in science was not only driven by my personal hopes; I was also delighted to be growing up in a nation whose strength, brilliance, and virtue were changing the course of history. The United States had defeated the demonic Nazis just eleven years before I was born. I was taught that we were holding the line against other people who intended to overrun the world if we weren't standing in their way. And we were destined for new forms of greatness through our national life.

This conviction—that a nation could live up to its ideals and be a force for good—was thrilling.

I was very young when John Kennedy became president—only four years old—but I could tell that a change had taken place in the whole country. The new president was energetic and funny and looked a bit like my father. I could tell that my father admired him. And this new president told us what I was already fully prepared to hear: that the country was going to do exciting, virtuous things, like sending astronauts to the moon.

Fifty years later, now that we have stopped launching space shuttles and seem to be abandoning the space age, it is hard to recapture how exciting rocket launches were for everyone. People paused at work to listen to the radio. Schools held special assemblies when the entire student body was marched into the auditorium to watch the launch on a single television. People would stare transfixed as the flight clock lost seconds and then would shout out the final countdown. Even on our small black-and-white televisions, the thundering climb into space made our hearts thump with excitement.

The space program got off to a fast start. Just a few months after Kennedy's inauguration, Alan Shepard became the first American to ride a flaming missile in a huge arc from Cape Canaveral to an ocean splashdown 116 miles away. When I was five and a half years old, John Glenn blasted off on February 20, 1962, and became the first American to orbit the earth.

More Mercury rockets took off, each containing one astronaut, until we moved to the Gemini program, in which two astronauts traveled together into space. The great objective, still years away, was the Apollo program, designed to send three astronauts a quarter million miles to the moon. John F. Kennedy's consistent message—that difficulties should intensify rather than weaken our commitment to boldness—became a window through which I began to see not only my own challenges but those of the nation and the world. The president made this clear in his initial announcement and in his subsequent comments about the space program. As the president said in Texas, "We choose to go to the moon in this decade . . . not because it is easy, but because it is hard, because that goal will serve to organize and measure the best of our energies and skills, because that challenge is one that we are willing to accept, one we are unwilling to postpone, and one which we intend to win."

Drawn by such daring visions, bubbling with curiosity, I yearned to know as much about the workings of the world as I could. My mother brought home stacks of brilliantly illustrated volumes from the Time-Life Science series that revealed some of the hidden mysteries and glories of our planet. I pored over volumes on the cell, the body, and the mind; on energy, matter, sound, and flight; on weather, planets, and space. Each photograph and diagram and paragraph reinforced what has become a fundamental part of my view of life: that we live in a magnificent universe with innumerable and beautiful secrets; that many of these secrets can be unlocked through the steady application of the human mind; and yet at the same time there will always remain an awe-inspiring complexity, vastness, and unknowable glory to creation. Those books, and the other materials that my parents carried home to feed my ravenous curiosity, helped me to peer past the edge of my wheelchair and bed, beyond the boundaries of our home and backyard, and into the mysteries that ruled everything from the tiniest cell in my body to the rhythm of galaxies in space.

*

While I was in elementary school, I missed weeks of classes at a time. At home, day after day I stared out my window, watching the trees sway in the wind as I waited interminably for my joints to heal. In the time before the Internet, the only sources of information were people, television, newspapers, books, and mail. I scoured them all. Whenever my parents invited other adults to dinner, I quizzed them about their lives. Our primitive television carried exactly seven channels, and I watched them all. I tried to make sense of the newspapers that arrived on our doorstep. I pulled every book I could reach off our shelves. I went through the mail like a detective, studying *TV Guide*, *Time*, and even the Sears catalogue with forensic care. When my parents finally bought an encyclopedia, I could not believe my good fortune—there were articles about everything, neatly bound in leather. My loneliness nurtured an insatiable desire to learn—about people, about places, and about the mysteries of life.

My parents did everything they could to feed this hunger. My sisters, Susanna and Elizabeth, helped me even more by providing companionship and balance in the struggle to grow up. I was far from a perfect child; I was often willful, noisy, impatient, and selfish. There was always the danger that my difficulties might drag me into a black hole of fury and self-pity.

I survived the long periods of convalescence by imagining the future. Having picked a moment or an event that I would like to see take place, I acquired the habit of working backward from that point through the steps that needed to take place so that I could get there. I lived through anticipation, and I was often disappointed, as bleedings and other problems forced the postponement and cancellation of dozens of longed-for events. With the encouragement of my parents, I steadily developed the rapid capacity to accept the new reality and establish a new goal. Through this process I slowly gained the upper hand over the soul-crushing emotion of regret.

As I observed others, I also inched away from my self-centered view. I realized that many, if not most, other people faced their own struggles. Passing in and out of hospitals, I saw children with far more serious physical problems than mine. Scanning the pages of the newspapers, I glimpsed the horrors of war and poverty and disease. Dipping more and more deeply into works of history and fiction, I imagined the hard lives that others had lived. I wanted to understand not just their ideas but their feelings, and this desire helped to move my curiosity past the mind and toward the heart. Slowly, as I did these things, a new emotional equation took hold: if my suffering prompted people to help me, then when others were suffering, perhaps I should try to help them.

The intuition started to influence my actions. I began to admire my parents and other adults when they took offense at injustice. I became incensed when I witnessed small acts of unfairness. Indeed, one of my earliest memories involves defying my elementary school classmates to defend a boy I did not even like.

I was in the first grade at the Valhalla Elementary School in Hartsdale, New York. One of my classmates brought his lunch every day in a brown paper bag. He was pudgy, abrasive, and loud—not someone I wished to get to know. His daily meal was dreary: a piece of bread, a stick of celery, an apple, and a hard-boiled egg. Every day at noon, when we arrived in the cafeteria, he would walk over to the lady at the cash register, reach into his pocket, and plunk down a nickel for a small container of milk.

Over time some of the boys in my class—the little lords of the lunchroom—began to object to the hard-boiled egg. His lunch was ridiculous, they said, snickering. It *smelled*. In a sense they were right—the eggs often did exude a slightly sulfurous odor that made me wonder how old they were. With each passing day, the egg boy's lunch became the focus of greater and greater ridicule. Finally, one day, when I was sitting at a nearby table, he sat down with some of these boys. When he pulled out his lunch, the cackling band pretended to gag. They punched him in the shoulder and demanded that he throw his whole lunch away. When he refused, they stood up, gathered their lunch trays, and marched as a group to another table on the other side of the lunchroom.

I watched him carefully. He slowly took another bite of the egg and wiped his eyes and nose on the back of his sleeve. With alarm, I realized that he was crying.

Up until that moment I had been an observer, eager to stay out of the line of fire, but his misery moved me. Without thinking, I picked up my tray, limped over to his table, and sat down beside him. He did not look at me or speak to me. For five awkward minutes we ate together in silence. From the corner of my eye I noticed the other boys giggling and smirking. Then, without a word, he and I stood up and went our separate ways.

In a movie version of this tale, he and I would have gone on to become the best of friends, but that did not happen. He remained loud and abrasive. His egg did smell pretty bad. And though I still didn't like him very much, at some elemental level, I had understood his feelings.

At other times I was only an observer of events that affected my parents and friends. During this period of his career my father worked for magazines such as the *Saturday Evening Post*. His editors would assign a story, he would spend weeks working on it, and at the last minute the piece would be blocked, leaving my father with a tiny "kill fee" instead of the more substantial payment he had expected and deserved.

On another occasion, my mother, still working part-time for Time-Life Books, had come up with the daring idea that they should produce a cookbook series. The editors asked for her ideas, so for weeks she pounded out suggestions, including proposed book outlines for two, the first on French provincial cooking and the second on Russian cuisine. The publishers loved the idea, and then my mother heard nothing more about it. Eventually she discovered that the whole project was being moved forward with substantial support from Time-Life Books.

The new editor in chief was a man without cooking experience. She rocketed into New York City and demanded to see the relevant executive.

"Why didn't you at least give me the chance to run this series?" she demanded.

The executive looked bemused.

"You couldn't possibly have thought that we would allow this series to be run by a *woman*, could you?" he asked her contemptuously.

When she came home crestfallen, I seethed.

*

At the age of eight, I learned that a large utility company, Consolidated Edison, had filed plans to build an immense hydroelectric storage facility on top of Storm King Mountain, a historic peak on the shore of the Hudson River in the Catskills, just a few miles north of West Point. The engineers planned to create a vast industrial storage tank into which water would be pumped at night, when electricity rates were low, and then that water would be released during the day to generate power through gravity-fed turbines. We had been on a school field trip to those breathtaking places—Storm King, Bear Mountain. I instinctively objected to the idea of destroying all of this to build a power plant.

Indeed, the battle over Storm King, which roiled the courts from the mid-1960s until 1980, was one of the earliest environmental legal fights—so early, in fact, that the term "environmentalism" did not exist, nor was the field of "environmental law" even recognized. At the time people who objected to the destruction of public beauty for private gain were known as "conservationists." Back then it was not a partisan issue; the nation's leading conservationists had included two Republican governors of New York, Theodore Roosevelt and Nelson Rockefeller. As the project advanced, citizens in the area, including the well-known Hudson Valley historian Carl Carmer and his wife, Betty, who lived in a huge and whimsical octagon-shaped house across the street from us, began to organize.

I wrote letters and drew pictures and mailed them off to the president of the United States and to national school newsletters, one of which printed them. The president sent me an autographed picture—which thrilled me—but did not comment on the dispute itself. As it turned out, the Scenic Hudson project, of which Storm King was a major component, became one of the most influential land-use cases in the country, establishing a host of precedents that launched the field of environmental law. The dispute took more than eighteen years to resolve before the courts finally ruled to block the power plant. The whole episode taught me that activists had to be committed for the long haul, because important battles often took years to be resolved.

*

To this day I wonder, how do we learn to speak up? How do we learn to find our voice and then to use that voice to open conversations, to raise questions, and, when necessary, to demand answers? We know that speech is fundamental to democracy, but why? Because the words we use, the reasons we offer, and the choices we make determine our future.

Many forces in the world would prefer us to remain mute. Speech is subversive, whereas silence, as the great Russian writer Aleksandr Solzhenitsyn said, is acquiescence. If we do not speak up in the face of injustice, we give others the right to decide not only what happens but to whom. Through speech we bind ourselves to each other and to our destiny. In silence we drift in both time and space.

To create community, to forge a bond in common, we must be able to communicate. When we understand one another's ideas and emotions, when we see into each other's lives, we span our differences and bring conscience and comfort to heal the brokenness of our world.

Somehow I figured this out at a fairly early age—as a gift from my artistic parents, as an insight handed to me through my own experiences, as a blessing from life itself. With each passing year I discovered more deeply that humans have both the definite duty and the glorious opportunity to cross over the divisions that naturally seem to separate us. Yes, we are all born into different moments and places, but our very individuality carries within it the mysterious key to a shared humanity. We speak separate languages, but our restless attempts to translate our thoughts into words and our words into deeds cause us to discover new points of contact and pathways of expression. We struggle in different moments and manners, and yet each apparent step into isolation can also create the opportunity for empathy.

Who was I, after all? Was I primarily a middle-class white American boy born into relative privilege compared to most children in the world? Or was I a pitiable child with a severe physical disability and a grim life expectancy? Did my future hold promise because of my mind or danger because of my body? Did my emerging fascination with American history and with the conservation of our environment mean that I was evolving into a conservative who disliked change or a progressive who embraced it? Was my love of reason, science, and astronomy at odds with my growing conviction that the universe was a place of overwhelming spiritual beauty?

When I reached adolescence I had an experience that vividly taught me how my own experiences, as dissimilar as they might seem to some, made me feel connected to others. As a young teenager, just after I had been released from extensive physical therapy in a hospital, I had the opportunity to tour Harvard College. The tour included a visit to the pool, where we came upon the swimming team at practice. We watched from the sidelines as the members of the Harvard team carved their way up and down the lanes as elegantly as dolphins. The coaches paced along the edges, blowing whistles and issuing instructions.

Watching them, I thought about a boy I had known in the hospital. Jamie had been born with osteogenesis imperfecta, also known as "brittle bone disease." His bones lacked a protein that maintained their structural integrity, so they snapped under the slightest trauma. Though only nine years old, he had already had twenty-seven operations. One of his legs had been amputated at the knee, the other at the ankle. He spent hours floating in whirlpool baths to strengthen his limbs and ease his pain.

His appearance was disturbing. When he sat on a chair, it looked as if he didn't have any legs at all. I think most people would at first have been horrified, as I was, yet as I came to know him, I grew to admire his humor and his courage. I encouraged him whenever I could. Sometimes I swam beside him in the pool, and whenever I did, I was grateful that I still had my legs and my strength.

While standing by the university pool, I thought about Jamie and about the Harvard men. I realized that the Harvard men would probably feel nothing but pity for Jamie, and Jamie would have trouble understanding the swimming team at all. And I realized that I belonged to both of their worlds—and to neither.

From then on, whenever I was in the pool myself, or taking on some other hard challenge, I returned to this core dream of bridging the gap between worlds. Whether in the swimming pool or during the daily challenges of life, I try to take a deep breath, drop my head below the surface, and push off toward the other side.

CHAPTER THREE

Black AND *White*

*I have struggled too long and too hard now to get rid
of segregation in public accommodations to end up at
this point in my life segregating my moral concerns . . .
Justice is indivisible. Injustice anywhere is a threat to
justice everywhere.*

—MARTIN LUTHER KING, JR.

Several years ago I received a Christmas gift in the mail
from my father: a framed photograph dated June 13,
1966. In the picture I am sitting in my lightweight aluminum
wheelchair on the white porch of our old house in Irvington,
New York. I look disheveled but happy. My white socks stick
out of my khaki pants, and I can see, even across the years,
that my left knee is swollen. I am wearing my absolute favorite
piece of clothing, a buckskin jacket with fringe on the shoulders—a style that I, along with millions of other little boys,
had adopted because of our enthusiasm for the Kentucky fron-
tiersman Davy Crockett. My right hand is raised to make an
enthusiastic point, and I am talking.

The person to whom my words are addressed is a tall, powerful African-American man who is balancing his massive body on a delicate wicker chair. We are only a few inches apart. He is leaning forward quietly, his arms resting on his knees, his right hand holding a glass of water. His head is turned sideways. His eyes reveal both curiosity and wariness as he studies my face. More than anything else, his expression says, "*I am listening to you.*" And looking at this moment frozen in time forty-five years ago, I feel a flush of pride, because he was so clearly honoring me with his attention and his respect.

The photograph now hangs in a hallway in my home in Massachusetts, and people are inevitably drawn to it. They look at it at first because they see that it is a picture of a young me during a hard time. Then they realize who the man beside me is. And they always turn to me and ask in astonishment, "Is that really Muhammad Ali?"

*

For me the picture captures a moment of deep change. Whenever I faced a lengthy period of recovery, my parents put out an appeal to their adult friends to come visit. Many thoughtful people stopped by. The person who brought the most energy and laughter, the person who swept aside any sadness that might be clinging to my heart, was our close friend Liz Parks. Born Elizabeth Campbell, the daughter of a well-known and successful cartoonist for *Esquire*, Liz had grown up largely in Switzerland, where her father had taken her to shield her from the tensions that they faced in the United States as a prosperous African-American family. Liz was a spectacular beauty, with the tall physique of a model and the sparkling eyes and elegant face of a princess. As a young adult she was drawn into the world of international high fashion. In her early twenties she met and married one of America's most famous photographers, Gordon Parks.

Gordon was in his fifties and had already lived a life of enormous challenge. He had started with a small camera and a fellowship from the Farm Security Administration to record the lives of African-Americans at work and at home in the ghetto. One of his most famous was a photograph of a maid with a broom and a mop standing in front of an American flag, which he called *American Gothic: Washington, D.C.* In 1948 a photo essay about a gang leader in Harlem won him a permanent position as a photographer and writer at *Life* magazine. Years later, speaking to a curator of an exhibit of his photos, Gordon explained the origin of his career. The camera, he said, "was my choice of weapon against what I hated most about the universe: racism, intolerance, poverty."

Liz visited frequently, and she always brought a typhoon of joy. I also loved visiting her house in White Plains during their many parties. They had a large swimming pool in the back. Gordon's twelve-cylinder dark green XK-E Jaguar crouched in the driveway, almost visibly breathing. In the living room, radiant light pulsed through huge plate-glass windows and a skylight to illuminate their paintings and pieces of sculpture. When they held a party, the whole house throbbed with enthusiasm and warmth. Music of all kinds, from classical to jazz, flowed continuously from speakers in every room. In warm weather—particularly during Fourth of July parties—children would come darting through the living room, dash into the backyard, and cannonball straight into the pool.

At their home we met musicians and journalists and painters and writers and rabble-rousers who discussed art and politics and told wonderful jokes. I thus grew up with a strange inversion of many young white Americans' experiences of race. Some white families feared African-Americans; most simply had little contact. Through Liz and Gordon, I obtained, within the limits of childhood, a new window into their particular American life, and I loved what I saw. Everything about my family—our clothes, our humor, our artwork, our car, our music—seemed pedestrian compared to Liz and Gordon's. I wanted to connect to their world—to *belong*.

In 1966 *Life* gave Gordon the assignment of photographing Muhammad Ali, the greatest boxer in the world, who was still known to many at the time as Cassius Clay. Gordon traveled everywhere with the charismatic Ali—to the gym for his workouts, to nightclubs for evening outings, to meals with his friends, and to meetings with advisers. After a week of taking pictures, it suddenly struck Gordon that in every one of these settings Ali had been surrounded entirely by a large entourage of black people. Gordon wondered what Ali's demeanor would be like—and what photographs might reveal—if he were to spend a few hours talking to a middle-class white family from the suburbs.

He and Liz conferred secretly with my parents. One spring evening my parents casually mentioned that Ali would be visiting the next day. I couldn't believe it. Throughout the evening they drilled me on how to address him.

"When he gets here," they said, "you say, 'How do you do, Mr. Ali?'"

"Right," I said.

"Mr. *Ali*," they insisted, "not Mr. Clay. You must not call him Mr. Clay."

"Mr. Ali," I repeated.

The next day I waited nervously on our porch, rolling aimlessly around in my wheelchair. Just about the time I couldn't stand it anymore, a huge eight-cylinder car came roaring up the driveway.

Mr. Ali, Mr. Ali, I repeated to myself silently.

The car pulled to a dramatic stop in front of our house. The twenty-four-year-old boxer, dressed in dark pants, a short-sleeved shirt, and elegant leather shoes, leapt out of the front passenger seat. He took our front steps two at a time; within a flash he was standing next to me with his hand out in a warm gesture of greeting.

"Hello, Mr.—" I started. That was as far as he let me get.

"Hello, kid!" he shouted exuberantly. "Do you know who I am?" Before I could answer he shouted, "I am the heavyweight champion of the world!"

I looked up at him, struck silent by his immense energy and mass. My parents invited him to move to the part of our porch that looked out over the river. He plunked down on our swing, but his 210-pound physique proved too much for the chains the chair was suspended from. As soon as he sat down, one of the chains snapped and sent him hurtling toward the ground. With instant reflexes he caught himself. We all erupted into elaborate apologies.

Gordon quickly smoothed over the situation and sat us all in a circle. The temperature was perfect; the sun glowed brightly through the leaves of our large elms and copper beech. My parents brought out tea and lemonade, and soon we were conversing while Gordon walked around silently, shooting photos from different angles while helping to move the conversation along. And somewhere in the midst of all of this, I opened up to Ali and began babbling away. It was at that second that Gordon caught the image.

When the time came for Ali to depart, I felt flooded with uncertainty about how to say goodbye. Before his arrival I had thought that I might ask him for his autograph, but when he stood up and reached out his hand to shake mine, I said the first thing that came into my mind.

"Mr. Ali, before you go, would you mind showing me your arm muscle?"

He smiled and crouched down beside me. He carefully pulled up the sleeve of his shirt and rolled it back over his shoulder. He slowly brought his entire arm to within inches of my face. And then, with a gleam of amusement, he flexed. I will never forget what it looked like. His arm seemed enormous, like the piston of a locomotive. And it was beautiful. His dark skin glistened in the light; his muscles curved magnificently into a sculpture that radiated power. I marveled that one human being could have that much force coiled in his body, ready for instantaneous use through a simple act of the mind.

"Wow," I said in a choked voice. "Thank you."

"That's okay, kid." He grinned and stood up. "You stay strong, all right?"

"All right," I said.

And then the scene reversed itself—the flurry of good-byes, the bounding down the steps, the spray of gravel as the car thundered out of the driveway. After he left I stared at the road for a long time.

A few weeks later my father and I were driving in a town near our home, past the local country club. It seemed lovely—it had a swimming pool, tennis courts, a pampered golf course, and an elegant clubhouse. Some of my friends from school had told me about this remarkable place, where people came together and ate lunch and played games and swam all afternoon. I envied them. We didn't have a swimming pool. I wondered if I could go there to meet other kids.

"So, Dad," I said enthusiastically, "why don't we join the country club?"

"No," he said emphatically.

"But why not? It looks great. Is it too expensive?"

"It is expensive, but that's not the reason," he said grimly.

I pressed on. "So what is the reason?"

He brought the car to a stop and turned to face me.

"Because I refuse to join a place that would never allow Liz and Gordon Parks to be members."

I was floored. What was he talking about?

"They can't be members because they live in another town?" I asked.

"No, Bobby," he said. "They cannot be members because they are black, and the country club does not admit black people."

"Because they are black?" I said stupidly.

"Yes," he said, "exactly."

*

This was not the first time I had heard of racism, but it stands out in my mind because it was so strikingly local and ordinary. My parents were journalists; we subscribed to many newspapers and magazines, and I had read about the stirrings in the South, the Freedom Rides, and the remarkable courage of Martin Luther King, Jr. We also had a family tie to these struggles. For decades my father's mother had been a ferocious activist in Nashville, Tennessee, fighting for a woman's right to vote and to choose. In her midfifties GrandMolly, as we called her, had become intensely involved in racial justice, so much so that the Ku Klux Klan burned a cross in her front yard. She was unafraid. When she examined the site the next day, she poked her toe in the ground. "Look at what they did to my petunias," she commented.

Later she participated in lunch counter sit-ins in her hometown. Those events took her all over downtown Nashville, including Harvey's, the city's largest and most elegant department store, where her husband was a senior manager. When his business colleagues asked why he couldn't control his wife, he told them to mind their own business. On another occasion GrandMolly invited an African-American friend to have lunch with her at a well-known segregated pancake house.

The nervous manager tried to escort them to the back of the restaurant, where they would not be observed. GrandMolly, always polite, stood her ground. She pointed to a table next to the big front window, where she and her companion would be visible from everywhere. "Young man, we are going to sit right there," she said. When they sat down, she unfolded her napkin and said to her companion, "I have always believed that in order to make change, we have to make ourselves seen."

*

I did not know what it meant to live as an African-American in a country consumed by race. At the same time, because of my experiences with hemophilia, I did know what it was like to walk into a room and to have people dismiss you in the space of a few seconds. I knew that my bandages and braces and wheelchair created a gap of anxiety or outright fear between me and those I met. I understood the desire to be accepted despite my appearance. And I knew how tiring and unfair it was to have to project warmth and confidence toward skittish strangers in order to induce them to accept one's elementary humanity.

Most of my days were spent crossing the long vistas of boredom and loneliness created by my slow recuperation from hundreds of joint bleedings. By this time we lived in a stately, crumbling Victorian house in Irvington, New York, that my parents had purchased in a fit of romance and financial folly. Known as Sunnybank, the hundred-year-old building needed endless repairs; for years we had to avoid slamming doors to avoid being doused with plaster dust from cracks in the ceilings above. The home exuded personality, though, likely a huge, shaggy old dog, and it sat on four acres filled with glorious trees—ramrod elms, soaring pines, and an immense 250-year-old copper beech that arched into the sky. Local historians said that Hessian troops—German mercenaries fighting against the American army during the revolution—had camped beneath its red canopy at the time of the Battle of White Plains, a detail that filled my mind with images during the long hours I stared out the window at its leaves and at the Hudson River in the distance.

For weeks on end, my primary instrument of propulsion was my wheelchair. It became an extension of my body. I knew just how fast I needed to be going to bump over the thresholds between rooms. I knew where and how to seize the doorjambs in a way that would allow me to slingshot around corners. I plucked the metal spokes of the wheels to create strangely attractive twelve-tone tunes. And I relieved the pressure on my back and legs by lifting the small front wheels off the floor and balancing on the two rear wheels, something I could do for hours on end.

I was able to move freely around this friendly ark of a house because of a large manual elevator hidden behind a door in the room where my father wrote. Designed like a huge dumbwaiter, the large wooden cage moved between the first and second floor through an ingenious system of counterweights and flywheels. I operated the device by yanking on thick ropes that opened the brakes and rotated the wheels to move the platform up and down. I was able to go downstairs for lunch, upstairs for the afternoon, and then downstairs for dinner, alternating venues as often as I could to alleviate the paralyzing tedium of convalescence.

As I headed into my teenage years, my circle of freedom and understanding expanded steadily. When I was eleven years old, a new treatment for hemophilia was invented: a high-potency form of Factor VIII that could be kept at room temperature and injected by the parents of boys with hemophilia or even the boys themselves. The availability of this new product was a godsend. It meant that bleedings could be treated quickly and effectively. With the support of these products I knew I might be able to build up the strength of my legs to the point where I could remove one, and then both, of my leg braces. The process was full of risk, because too much stress could plunge me back into weeks or months of incapacity. The reward, however, was potentially miraculous.

I remember one afternoon in particular when I was given a small taste of the freedom that might lie ahead. I was sitting on the back steps of our house, looking at a tire swing that my father had suspended from a maple tree. I had just removed my braces and was wondering how many steps I might be able to take without them. I realized that though I had often watched my sisters at play on the swing, I had never been on it. Somehow I limped and stumbled across the yard until I could grab the swing with my hands. I tucked my legs through the center and began to glide back and forth, side to side, in great swooping figure eights. As I moved through the air, I felt a rush of liberation. The speed, the windy air, the circular motion, were all new to me. They instantly evoked all the things I could not do: run, skate, or fly. As I swirled around I was experiencing life in a new manner, through the eyes and body of someone who was no longer tied to the ground.

It was an illusion, in many ways, but it gave me a foretaste of what would happen if I could remain disciplined and break free from the devices that tied me down. In the moments I rode on the tire swing, I experienced the exhilaration of motion, the joy of a new form of dance, both physical and spiritual, that lay just ahead. And within months, supported by the new medical technologies and motivated by this new vision of freedom, I finally took the braces off.

Yet I could not throw them away. The metal bars and leather straps and carefully handmade buckles had been part of my life for too long. Even though I had feared and resented them, they had given me what little mobility I had had over many years.

They now lie in a large plastic box in the cool darkness of a small room in our basement. Every few years I am down there looking for Christmas ornaments or old books and I come across them. When I open the lid, they always shock me, and it is all I can do not to weep.

*

In the fall of 1968 my parents moved our whole family overseas to the magnificent city of Paris. They had completed their work on my father's first book, *Nicholas and Alexandra*, and with its publication and overnight transformation into a bestseller we suddenly had the resources to do new things. My mother, who had been born in the United States to Swiss parents, was especially eager for us to learn French so that we could forge ties with our relatives.

To move my parents, my two sisters, a babysitter, and me, along with all of our luggage for a year, we decided to take the S.S. *France,* one of the last of the great fleet of transatlantic ocean liners that went back and forth every week. As we stood on the deck and felt the huge vessel pulling away from Manhattan, my mother leaned over and reminded me of the conversations we had had when I had been frightened, strapped to the hospital bed many years before. "I told you that someday we would go to Paris," she said, her eyes sparkling.

Though our original plan was to go for twelve months, we ended up remaining for the next four years. The first year Susanna and I attended the Ecole Bilingue, which accepted both English- and French-speaking students. I was placed in a small classroom of French beginners who were twelve or thirteen years old. Within a few days I discovered that Paris worked its magical effects on people of every age.

We eventually moved to one of the oldest sections of Paris, the Marais, and lived in a four-hundred-year-old apartment building. We had a small garden in the back, and just over the garden wall were the barracks of the Garde Republicaine, a cavalry unit of the French army much like the British Royal Horse Guards. The president of France often used this regiment, in full dress uniform, swords drawn, to welcome foreign heads of state or to escort him in parades. Every morning as we drank our coffee and prepared to go to school, we could hear the clip-clop of their chestnut horses as the guards practiced their maneuvers, often combined with the brilliant harmonies of their trumpets.

Coming from America, we were captivated by everything that was different. Many of the city's streets revealed the capital city's preoccupation with two of its major pursuits: fashion and food. I was mesmerized by the endless number of places to eat. Every street was lined with bistros and cafés, with patisseries (selling pastries and ice cream), boulangeries (selling all the popular forms of bread and many other prepared foods), and fromageries (cheese stores). Specialty stores for fish, meat, fruit, vegetables, and wine squeezed into tiny spaces next to each other from one side of the city to the other. At that time there were few supermarkets and the refrigerators in most apartments were tiny, so most people bought something fresh for their meals every day. When they didn't want to eat at home, people sat at tiny outdoor tables on the sidewalks of the boulevards and ordered food and drink from well before breakfast until long after midnight.

After we spent a year in a supposedly bilingual school, where, unfortunately, we learned very little French, my parents transferred us to a new school, the Collège Sévigné, on the Left Bank. The experience plunged me into yet another setting in which I was made aware of my differences from the community around me. I was an American in a school full of French children, and a boy in a sea of girls.

Established in 1880 as the first nondenominational school for young women in France, the Collège Sévigné had endured for nearly ninety years as a single-sex facility until the turbulent events of 1968, when an explosion in French society pitted leftist university students against a conservative government and a tough police force. The crisis led to months of anarchy in the schools and factories, and thousands of other institutions simply stopped functioning. Seeking relief from the chaos, parents clamored for the schools where they had enrolled their daughters to admit their sons as well. I entered in the first coeducational class. In my eighth-grade class there was only me and a French boy named Jean-Yves Grindel with twenty-six girls.

It was not easy to win acceptance in such a setting, particularly since we were all skidding into puberty. Teenage Parisian girls, like their counterparts around the world, showed little interest in boys their own age. The thrill in their lives came from high school boys, even college students, who arrived at the end of the school day on their buzzing mopeds, their long dark hair and scarves trailing in the wind, cigarettes hanging lazily from their mouths. My female classmates would hop on the back of these machines, wrap their arms around the waist of the boy in front of them, and go speeding off with the sound of squealing tires and laughter. Sometimes I would spot them in nearby cafés, smoking and drinking red wine with their wire-thin admirers, while I sighed, reshouldered my book bag, and trudged home.

Though I was barred from these emerging romantic encounters, some girls still reached across the cultural divide to include me. They found my strange accent, my clumsy verbal mistakes, and even my unusual medical problems interesting. Their affection was similar to what one would show to a pet. It didn't help that in France my name, Bobby, was the stereotypical name for a cute little dog. At the same time, there was an element of mercy in their efforts of inclusion. Some girls, recognizing that I had absorbed almost nothing of what was said in class for the first few weeks, cornered me in the corridors, at lunch, or in study hall to offer emergency tutorials before the next class.

At the time, the French national system of education, designed by Napoleon to create a uniform national standard of excellence, thrived on ranking, ordering, grading, and excluding. There was no sense that a child—especially a middle-school child—should be offered flexibility and room to grow. The goal of the system was to sort children quickly into the areas in which they would best serve the state. By the time most children were fifteen, they had been classified into iron categories that determined what they would be allowed to study, what universities they would be permitted to attend, and thus what careers they would be able to pursue—elite careers in science or government for those with the best scores, teaching careers in the humanities for the next ranks, and trades for everyone else. Once these decisions had been made, there was virtually no chance to alter the outcome.

To speed the process of sorting, schools measured, graded, recorded, and finally published results for every student by class, subject, and age group. Class rankings were announced publicly after every test, and in every subject every six weeks. Grades were based on a scale of 1 to 20. Class participation and deportment counted for a great deal. Teachers enforced discipline by handing out extra zeros, which arbitrarily lowered one's score and rank for the month.

The system reeked of bias and whim. "Do you want to know what kind of grades you can expect from me?" one teacher asked us early in the year. "Here is my scale. Twenty is reserved for Almighty God. Nineteen is for the original author of the passage, such as Racine or Corneille. Eighteen is for the greatest scholar in the world. Seventeen would be for me. Your scores will all fall underneath—in most cases very far underneath." Under these circumstances a student was considered a genius of the first order if she or he received a 15. Most students felt thrilled to pocket a 12.

Like every Western society in the late 1960s, France seethed with turmoil. There were so many strikes and demonstrations by workers and students that the French government deployed a specially trained and brutal group of riot police, known as the Companies Républicaines de Sécurité, or CRS, virtually every week. The CRS wore black helmets, tall boots, and dark blue uniforms specifically designed for street battle; they carried truncheons and plastic shields. I routinely discovered on my way to school that CRS trucks had cordoned off some section of Paris. One morning my municipal bus became stuck in the middle of a fierce demonstration; I watched as demonstrators and CRS officers flailed away at each other on the street corners. At one point two CRS officers grabbed a young female demonstrator. One of the men held her arms behind her back while the other deliberately stomped sideways on her ankle, breaking it. They then dropped her on the ground and fled.

*

There were also many good sides of French society. Like all the other countries in Europe, France had emerged from World War II with a deep commitment to provide health care to every citizen in the country. Unlike the United States, with its haphazard and unjust system of free-market insurance, France believed that everyone deserved health care as a right and created an interlocking system of national and private delivery and payment systems. To our surprise, my parents discovered that we were eligible for French health insurance, even though we were only residents, not citizens. Apparently the government considered it unthinkable that a child with a severe illness such as mine would not be treated on French soil simply because he or she had the wrong passport. In part because of this government policy, which gave me unlimited access to key blood products whenever I needed them, I experienced greater and greater freedom from bleeding at the same time that I was going through puberty and seeking more independence. Though I still had terrible problems from time to time, I was eventually able to stabilize my condition enough to travel on the subway at will and explore distant parts of the city for many hours on end.

I also wanted to bring greater freedom to my classmates at school. I felt that the students lacked a voice and a venue in which to discuss the changes they wanted to see. The solution, I decided, was obvious: a school newspaper! When I proposed the concept to my friends, they all thought it excellent—and completely hopeless. Students expressing their own ideas? *Impossible*.

I made an appointment with the formidable head of the school, known as Mme. la Directrice, and appeared at the appointed hour wearing a tie and carrying a pile of carefully prepared notes. She was a tiny woman who dressed entirely in black and whose silver hair was pulled back in a bun that suggested a helmet. She listened to me with a furrowed brow; I could not tell whether I was making progress or digging myself into deep trouble. Finally, at the end, she paused for a long time and then said she would consider it. The next day she called me back in, and to my surprise, she said that she would approve it as long as she could review the document before it was printed.

The whole project quickly became an example of the adage "Be careful what you wish for." A handful of overworked students had to solicit, write, edit, illustrate, type, and mimeograph the articles. After six weeks of intense labor, my classmates and I brought out the first—and, it turned out, the only—newspaper in the ninety-year history of the school.

We also took on the rampant problem of cheating. Because of the emphasis on memorization and grades, students tried every trick they could think of to give themselves an advantage. They wrote notes on their hands or on tiny pieces of paper that they concealed in their jewelry. They sat next to each other and copied each other's exam papers. In many cases the teachers simply turned a blind eye; students often brought their textbooks into the testing room and secretly balanced them on their knees just below the level of the tabletop, so they could copy directly from them.

When I brought it up, everyone agreed that this was a

serious problem. I quickly realized that their concern was not enough. The students did not want to stop doing it, and the teachers did not want to admit that it was taking place, and so nothing happened. My efforts at organizing foundered. From this I learned a lesson about the special challenge of trying to create change when there is no constituency to support it.

*

The longer I was in France, the more I came to admire the United States. Part of it was the longing that comes over every expatriate to return to his or her country. At one point I experienced such longing for America that it influenced a major purchase. I had accumulated a small amount of money from odd jobs and allowance, and I was thinking about purchasing a guitar or a tape recorder. I went to a French music store and noticed a long row of banjos lining the top of the wall.

"What are those?" I asked.

"That one is a six-string banjo, tuned like a guitar," said the young man. "And that one is a four-string jazz banjo."

"And what's that one?" I asked, pointing to the last one in the row.

"That's the five-string *American* banjo," he said.

I bought it on the spot.

"How can I learn to play it?" I asked, a little late.

He shrugged his shoulders. Then his eyes lit up and he dashed into a room behind the counter. I heard him tossing papers and books around. A few minutes later he emerged with a mimeographed copy in English of *How to Play the 5-String*

Banjo, by Pete Seeger. I went home happy and locked myself in my room for the better part of a week. I have been playing ever since.

Thus, looking at American culture from a distance, I came to see its good qualities. Though my family and I opposed the Vietnam War, I grew tired of listening to constant criticism of American policy. I became particularly incensed when people thought that the United States was the only country in the world that had a problem with racism. Once, over lunch, an aging woman whose only job was to sit at the top of the stairs and shout at children to slow down came over to speak to me. She launched into a lengthy attack on America's appalling treatment of its minority citizens. I listened for a while.

"But don't you believe, Madame, that France has its own problems with race?" I said. "I see Africans sweeping the streets and Algerians working construction, but in no other jobs. Perhaps the French people have their own difficulties with race?"

"Oh no, *pas du tout*!" she exclaimed. "We are not racists in any way! We even let them be policemen!"

*

Living abroad also brought us into contact with an endless string of fascinating people from all over the world who filed through our home and told their stories. One of the universal themes was the escape from tyranny. Sitting in Europe, barely two decades away from World War II and only a few hundred miles from the military power of the Soviet Union and the Warsaw Pact, we became keenly aware of the human dimension of the struggle for human rights.

Our family was deeply involved in Russian history and contemporary Russian life. My father set to work on what turned into a ten-year project of writing a biography of Peter the Great. My mother wrote a series of essays and translations of Russian poetry, printed in both Russian and English. It was published in 1972 as *The Living Mirror: Five Young Poets from Leningrad*. During her many trips to Russia my mother had also fallen in with a circle of painters, dancers, and other artists. She began to collect their stories and, in modest amounts, their works, smuggling them out among her clothes.

We heard at first hand about Soviet brutality against those the state considered intellectually or politically dangerous. When the Soviet secret police suspected that one of our friends and one of Russia's great character dancers, Sasha Mintz, wanted to leave Russia, they sent thugs who beat him and broke his collarbone. We were horrified, for we knew that such an attack could easily have ended his career. My parents also fought for years on behalf of the ballet couple Valery and Galina Panov. Though Valery was one of the greatest dancers in all Russia, he was largely unknown in the West, because he had been allowed to perform only a single time in New York. When he applied to emigrate to Israel, he was fired and exiled to a distant rural town; his wife, Galina, also a dancer, was pressured to divorce him; and he lived with the daily fear of violence and assassination. After many years he was released, but only after my parents and hundreds of other supporters in the West held protests and pressured the Soviet Union to stop its destruction of this exceptional artist.

That single success did little to alter our disgust with Soviet human rights violations and hypocrisy. I learned through these experiences that the crime of brutalizing citizens required no particular political label. It did not matter whether the government was identified as left-wing or right-wing; dictators were dictators. They needed to be opposed no matter what the political excuses for their behavior. Stories of persecution and brutality arrived almost daily in the mail or over the ancient black telephone that sat on the oval table near the window overlooking the courtyard with its peaceful trees.

*

One day when I was fifteen, our friend Phyllis Glaeser asked if we would like to come that evening to see the rough cut of a documentary by a friend of hers. In the small screening room we met a quiet and intense black director named Nelson ("Nana") Mahomo. The film, called *Last Grave at Dimbaza*, depicted the brutal system of racial segregation that governed a country I had never heard of—South Africa. The focus of the film was the policy of resettlement, under which black citizens, particularly women and children, who had moved to towns and squatter camps near South Africa's major cities were forcibly relocated to distant spots in their "homelands"—in fact, little more than bleak, waterless dumping grounds. The South African minister of justice argued that the breakup of families was justified because "black workers must not be burdened with superfluous appendages like women and children." The resulting misery, poverty, malnutrition, and disease decimated the population, so much so that in some parts of the country only half the babies lived past the age of five.

Apartheid was a system specially designed for the twentieth century and aggressively defended as a positive good. It was administered by an intelligent, mechanized modern government controlled by an all-white political group known as the National Party. In addition, this government frequently proclaimed itself a democratic ally of the United States, something that American presidents seemed to tolerate. And judging from the numerous shots of American corporate facilities that popped up throughout the film, the United States apparently had extensive and unapologetic commercial arrangements with the white rulers of this regional power on the tip of the great continent.

The message of the film struck me powerfully. What impressed me even more, however, was Nana Mahomo's attitude. While we fidgeted in our seats, flinching at the grotesque truths that the film implacably laid before us, Nana sat quietly. When the movie was over and the small audience asked him questions, he answered with an intensity both quiet and strangely majestic.

Though he was reluctant to talk about his own experience, we gradually pieced together his story. He was a member of the Pan Africanist Congress (PAC), a vigorous rival to the African National Congress. On March 21, 1960, seeking to spark a national uprising against white rule—and to gain the upper hand over the ANC—the PAC called for a general strike. Robert Sobukwe, the head of the PAC, personally asked Mahomo to leave the country the day before in order to serve as an ambassador extraordinaire, ready to explain the new regime to foreign governments and to negotiate relationships for the new government among the family of nations. Instead, the uprising failed. Not enough people learned of it in time. Those who did congregate met a murderous South African police and military.

In the town of Sharpeville, white forces fired rifles, pistols, and machine guns directly into a packed crowd of protesters. Sixty-nine fell dead, including more than a dozen women and children—many shot in the back—in what became known as the "Sharpeville massacre." Robert Sobukwe, in an act of brash courage, turned himself in to the police for violating the official "pass laws"; they happily arrested him and jailed him for the rest of his life. His colleagues were hunted down, imprisoned, or shot. Mahomo, watching these events from abroad, realized that he was now completely cut off from everything and everyone to which he had devoted his life.

For the next decade Mahomo traveled and spoke about the injustices unfolding in his home country. He encountered wide disbelief among his audiences. Beginning in 1969 he and a group of British film students spent three years getting various friends to obtain and smuggle out clandestine footage. He maintained his composure and resolve through innumerable setbacks. Slowly he assembled enough images and money to craft a full documentary. He knew that he faced potentially deadly retaliation. South African secret agents regularly assassinated "Communists" and "terrorists" all over the world.

The experience opened my eyes even more to the reality of oppression and tyranny. It was not just the people of the Soviet Union or Communist China who endured mindless cruelty from their own governments; governments that cloaked themselves in the language of democratic rights were also guilty. Nana's patience and reserve introduced me to the realities of South Africa but also showed me how raw outrage was not enough to create change. The pursuit of lasting justice requires a depth of commitment that transcends the emotion of the moment. I could see that real leaders had to learn how to live with a slow, deep, burning passion for justice that was both a source of motivation and a wound. One never knew whether one's actions would really have effect, whether one would live to see the transformation for which one longed. The dedication itself—ringed and supported with a hope and trust in the direction of history—had to be enough.

For some, the burden was too much or the answers never came. For others, including Nana, the frustration was rewarded with occasional moments of triumph that helped refuel the effort. A few months after we saw the film, *The Last Grave at Dimbaza* was shown on national television in the United States and won an Emmy. The debate over America's political and commercial entanglement with apartheid intensified. New opponents of apartheid appeared among student, religious, and civil rights groups. And Nana went back to many more years in his restless and sometimes controversial search for political allies, personal advancement, ideological justification, and fundamental change in the country from which he was barred. After a few conversations, I never saw him again.

But I never forgot him.

CHAPTER FOUR

In AND *Out*

Few are willing to brave the disapproval of their
fellows, the censure of their colleagues, the wrath of
their society. Moral courage . . . is the one essential,
vital quality for those who seek to transform a world
which yields most painfully to change.

—ROBERT F. KENNEDY

In September 1972 we left Paris for good and returned to the rambling old house in Irvington. I was sixteen and enrolled in a nearby high school, Hackley School. Because of the intensity of French education, I found that I was a full year ahead of my peers, so I was bumped up into my senior year. I did my best to stay above water academically. I also continued to be interested in human rights. I learned of Vladimir Bukovsky, a Russian neurophysiologist who had been arrested in the 1960s. The Soviet police sent him to one of their many psychiatric prisons on the grounds that anyone who opposed the Soviet Union's policies must by definition be mentally ill, since the Soviet system was self-evidently the best in the world.

Once locked away, the prisoners faced solitary confinement, physical restraint, forced injection with drugs, beatings, starvation, and death. In the face of such horrific treatment, Bukovsky proved particularly courageous. His first crime had been organizing a poetry reading; for that he was sent to psychiatric prison for three years. The second time he led a gathering to protest the arrest of other dissidents, and he was again jailed. In 1971 he secretly conveyed 150 pages of documents about the Soviet abuse of psychiatry to the West. He then received what was likely to be a permanent sentence. From the Soviet government's standpoint, he had been crushed; once he was out of sight, they assumed he would disappear from everyone's mind.

Amnesia is a tool of injustice, and memory is one of the most important means to combat it. Bukovsky might be sitting in some hidden prison, and I might only be a high school student worrying about grades, SAT's, and girlfriends, but I was determined to play some tiny part in keeping his name and his cause from fading away. And so I launched my own haphazard campaign to free him. I persuaded my classmates to write letters to the Soviet ambassador. I drafted petitions and took them whenever my parents attended gatherings of other activists.

Even though I doubt anything I did benefited Bukovsky directly, the process became something of a spiritual discipline for me. I found a large picture of him and posted it in my room, and later in my college dormitory. I glanced at it every morning when I left and every evening when I returned. It served as a visual tuning fork to keep me from being distracted. It reminded me that every day I lived in freedom, he languished in prison. In this manner, he never became invisible. He was a living being, who woke each morning and shivered with cold and reached out every day to touch his prison bars. My actions might have seemed pointless to some, but they were not worthless to me.

Nor, in the end, to him. Many years later, after he had been freed and when he made his first trip to the United States, I met him. I had the chance to shake that long-imprisoned hand— and he thanked me.

*

I finished Hackley School in the spring of 1973, earlier than I had expected, and I decided to take an extra year before going to college. I worked a few odd jobs and used the money to take flying lessons. Looking for something to do in the spring, I sent out dozens of letters and was lucky enough to be hired as an intern for U.S. Senator Henry M. "Scoop" Jackson. Jackson had been elected to Congress in 1940. When war broke out, he enlisted in the military, but President Roosevelt sent word to the Pentagon to kick out all the congressmen and send them back to their jobs. Jackson was an old-school Democrat, a New Deal progressive who had cautious foreign policy views. In some circles he was viewed as a hawk on Vietnam, but he was also one of the leading proponents of human rights in the Soviet Union and around the world.

I was installed as the most junior possible intern in the

Senate Permanent Subcommittee on Investigations, a roiling bullpen of investigators presided over by the great foreign policy expert Dorothy Fosdick. My job was to make photocopies, get coffee, attend hearings, take notes, and just soak up as much of the culture of the U.S. Senate as possible.

It was a turbulent time, because just upstairs, in the Russell Senate Caucus Room, the brilliant lights of live television were shining down on the hot and hapless witnesses who were appearing before the Senate select committee on Watergate. Occasionally I got into the office early enough to get a seat at the very back of the room, where I watched the great crocodile of the Senate, Sam Ervin of North Carolina, preside over the tawdry story that was unfolding in front of him with the skill of a wily country judge. Day after day, week after week, month after month, the hearings went on, as it became clear that the culture of corruption in American politics had stained more deeply than anyone had previously been willing to admit. My rosy and enthusiastic view of the glories of democracy began to fade as I listened to men and women who worked for President Nixon testify to a long litany of lying, cover-ups, bribery, and other crimes. It all came to a head just as I was leaving Washington, when it became clear that the president of the United States himself had been part of the conspiracy. Impeachment proceedings jumped forward, and in August 1974 the president dramatically resigned.

My role in Washington did not end at that moment, however, because I became involved in a project that took me back for the two following summers. Senator Jackson had become increasingly interested in the way large companies traded raw materials through international markets, rewarding some and punishing others as a way to increase their profits. He was in the midst of using the staff skills in the Investigations Subcommittee to probe the dealings of international oil companies.

When I went back to work for him in the summer of 1975, I became interested in the global trade in blood products, and I researched how products such as Factor VIII were collected, how they were made, and where they were sold. As I learned more and more about the industry, I became alarmed about how these firms were collecting blood from the poorest, most vulnerable, and often least healthy people in the world, from impoverished Nicaraguan peasants to skid-row bums in American cities. I learned that even though the products were thought to be infected with hepatitis (we only knew about hepatitis A and B then), they were being marketed aggressively in Europe and elsewhere as the most advanced form of treatment for hemophilia and other bleeding disorders. They were in fact very convenient for someone who could get a needle into his own veins, yet they came from a system so blinded by the desire for profit that the growing dangers of contamination were ignored.

I persuaded Senator Jackson and some of his staff that there were serious questions which deserved examination. Senator Jackson eventually sent an official letter to all the major pharmaceutical companies that made blood products, asking them for more detailed information about the supply, manufacture, safety, pricing, and distribution of their products.

We received two kinds of answers. Some companies sent us boxes and boxes crammed with promotional brochures, irrelevant memos, shipping manifests, factory manuals, and other loosely related material. The other companies sent us a single-page letter, which, in not very subtle but still highly legal terms, told Senator Jackson to go to hell.

Jackson was not happy, and his team discussed pushing the investigation to a higher level of intensity. They began to consider issuing subpoenas and holding hearings in order to get to the bottom of what was going on. This process unfolded over many months. We made progress, but the staff became distracted because Senator Jackson was preparing to run for president of the United States in 1976. At the same time, they kept me working on the project.

One morning I received a surprise phone call from the minority counsel, the head of the Republican staff of the committee. He wanted to meet with me personally—now. I was perplexed. Senior Senate staff members of one party do not usually summon interns from another party to hold urgent private meetings. I mentioned this to my immediate boss at the time, and he said, "Go see what he wants."

I walked through the immense hallways of the Russell Senate Office Building, passing office after office of different senators, with their great mahogany doors and American and state flags standing majestically in the hallways. My feet clicked and echoed on the vast marble floor. When I reached my destination, I was ushered immediately into the minority counsel's office. He was seated behind his desk with his hands folded.

"Sit down," he said.

I did.

"I have asked you to come here because I understand that Senator Jackson is considering issuing subpoenas in the pharmaceutical investigation."

I said nothing.

"I have consulted with the ranking minority member of the subcommittee, Charles Percy, and he has a problem with that. Specifically, he has a problem with *you*."

I was shaken. Percy was one of the most famous senators in the country, widely considered a decent man and a Republican moderate. He was also from Illinois, the home of most of the pharmaceutical manufacturers. The minority counsel continued with an edge to his voice.

"We believe that your personal medical situation makes it completely inappropriate for you to be involved in any investigation of this industry. So we have decided that we will consider supporting this investigation only if you withdraw from it. You must recuse yourself immediately and completely. If you don't, we will block any subpoena. So it's your choice— the investigation either stops here or you quit and give it the chance to go forward." He paused for effect and then waved his hand. "Now you can go."

I walked back through the long corridors in shock, realizing that I had just been exposed to my first direct case of political hardball. When I returned, I told the majority counsel, who was furious. Together we went to Senator Jackson, who was equally angry that the Republicans had called me in private. Jackson was a realist, and he said to me, "Bob, you know this presidential thing is coming up, so I would have a lot of trouble forcing this through right now. If I am elected president, you will come see me at the White House and we will use my authority to find out what is going on. And if I lose, I will return to the Senate and we will crack this resistance right here."

I left his office and thought, Well, something is going to happen; there is just going to be a delay. But Jackson did not win the nomination—that went to Jimmy Carter—and I gave up my position in the Senate. When Jackson returned to the Senate, he was swamped with foreign policy problems. A few years later he died suddenly, at the age of seventy-one. The subpoenas, the investigation, and the hearings never took place.

Between Watergate, the endless agony of the Vietnam War, and the crushing of the pharmaceutical investigation, I decided that I had seen enough. I was finished with politics.

*

In the fall of 1974 I had enrolled as a freshman at Princeton University, a bastion of dazzling opportunity and privilege. My father, my uncle, my doctor, and my godfather had all earned scholarships from Tennessee to attend Yale, and my initial idea had been that this was where I might go. When I applied to Yale, however, I encountered some harsh physical realities. Though I was now able to walk without braces, my knees remained weak. I still had joint bleedings, which would regularly confine me to a wheelchair for a week or more. Seen through this lens, the Yale campus presented many barriers. It had been built with the assumption that every student would be perfectly mobile. Classrooms could be reached only at the top of long stairways in buildings that were far apart. The mostly Gothic design of the dormitories and refectories, bunched together in "colleges," meant that everyone had to navigate through a maze of difficult hallways and stairs. The architects seemed to have been committed to the idea that every passageway or building entrance required at least three randomly placed steps.

Moreover, Yale was in the middle of a city, New Haven, so the students traveling between class and college activities had to cross urban streets all day long. Cities at that time did not build curb cuts to allow wheelchairs to roll smoothly from sidewalk to crosswalk. As I looked around, my heart sank when I realized that I could easily be confined to a small room, missing events and classes, forcing classmates to carry cold plates of food from distant dining rooms back to my point of incarceration. And while the admissions office expressed concern about my problems, no one was all that eager to discuss or to solve them. The Americans with Disabilities Act had not yet passed the Congress, and indifference or insensitivity toward people with disabilities was still more the rule than the exception.

This was in direct contrast to Princeton. After I was admitted, the admissions office designated a specific person to help me resolve each difficulty. Though the campus was self-contained, it was still hard for me to navigate on foot. We hit on the solution of obtaining a small electric cart that would transport me from class to class. The university promised to put in external electric plugs anywhere I needed them—outside my dorm room, the dining room, and the major classroom buildings—so I could charge the cart as necessary. If I had a bleeding and needed care, I would be permitted to enroll directly in the school infirmary, without the usual medical review, so that I could have a quiet place to recover, three meals a day, and easy access to friends who would drop by with my assignments. The university offered to exempt me from the lottery for dorm rooms so that I could find the right room. If I experienced a lasting problem, the authorities said, they would even reschedule my class discussion groups to meet on the first floor so I did not have to climb stairs to attend.

Of course the academic opportunities at both institutions were superb. I understood the tremendous privilege that each represented. Change was rippling through both universities and many other elite institutions as they tried to find a way to balance their traditional exclusivity with their desire to be more diverse. Every college in the country, including the Ivy League schools, was trying to figure out how to boost their enrollment of students disadvantaged by race or class and give them the support that would guide them toward success. Yale and Princeton had also just fought major battles with their own conservative alumni, who did not want them to admit women. The first women at Princeton had arrived only five years before I enrolled, and the first full class that included women had just graduated.

Schools were new to the issue of how—or even whether—to support students with disabilities. For some schools, the idea of admitting students with disabilities seemed perhaps to contradict the idea of gathering together "well-rounded" participants who were fully equipped to compete and to succeed. Subtle differences in attitude led to huge differences in outcomes. One school, with the best of intentions, told me, in essence, that it would be content for me to come as long as *I* could conform to *its* reality. The other university reversed the equation, saying, "We know that we need to change and that we have not been welcoming to some people in the past. Our goal is for you to feel fully included and to have everything you need while you are here to succeed." In response, I gratefully picked Princeton.

I arrived on campus and plummeted into the whirlwind of freshman year. During the first few weeks I was ecstatically happy. The campus was remarkable, but my new friends proved the greatest asset of all. Gathered from around the country and the world, representing innumerable backgrounds, drawn by different interests, they were electrifying. Given their array of talents, I also felt queasy. The man who became my first roommate and best friend was named Stephen Chanock. From Washington, he was tall and handsome, with a tousle of curly black hair. He was a swimmer who had competed nationally. He had scored higher than anyone I had ever met on all of his advanced placement tests. He was a math whiz. He played the piano beautifully and planned to be a composer. Or a doctor. Or both.

My mild anxieties did not prevent me from doing what all

freshmen do: I overcommitted. I signed up for a broad range of courses, including first-year Russian, which met twice a day. I attended meetings and poked my nose into campus politics. Over dinner my friends and I engaged in long philosophical conversations in which we all made firm pronouncements on topics about which we were completely uninformed. I even went to see the coach of the swimming team, who was famous for being gruff. I told him that I was slow and often had trouble walking but that I wanted to work out in the practice pool near the swim team.

"I don't care about your performance," he said, "I care about your commitment. If you are in the water every day at exactly seven A.M. and then again at two-thirty P.M. and you stay for the full workout both times, you can participate."

For the next nine months I kept up the schedule. When I returned the following fall, the coach handed me the team roster with a silent, knowing smile. I scanned the list and realized with astonishment that he had listed me on the swim team. The idea was absurd—I was the slowest swimmer in the group and could not really compete at the varsity level—but he had recognized my tenacity. I have rarely been as proud.

*

In my room, and whenever I left the campus, I always carried a small canvas bag that I referred to as my "shot bag." It contained everything I needed to treat my hemophilia on short notice: 23g butterfly needles, 30cc syringes, medical tape, alcohol prep pads, bottles of sterile water, tourniquet, ace bandage, ice bag, and small boxes of the critical freeze-dried Factor VIII concentrate on which my body depended if my joints started to bleed. I didn't take it to class or to meals, but otherwise it went with me everywhere: on every car ride or trip, to every off-campus meeting or dinner party or movie; on visits, on vacation, and on airplanes. It was not life-threatening for me to be without it, but whenever a joint started swelling—which usually happened without warning—a delay in mixing up and injecting the Factor VIII could mean the difference between a few hours and many weeks of painful limitations. Though I rarely thought about the bag when I was carrying it, I instantly knew when it was missing.

It was my chain and my lifeline for decades. I had had to administer infusions of Factor VIII as often as five times a week since I was twelve years old. No matter where I was, no matter how late at night or how inconvenient the moment, I had to stop whenever I felt a slight swelling and slip away to some private place where I mixed up the medications, strapped a tourniquet on my arm, and then inserted a needle into a vein. I had performed such injections in every conceivable venue: at parties, in airplane bathrooms, in train compartments, under the beam of a flashlight on camping trips. Even as my veins became filled with scar tissue and the skin on the surface turned an unappealing shade of blue, I rarely missed. My friends gradually became accustomed to this peculiarity, and some of them were even willing to witness the infusions.

The medications were enormously expensive, and I lived with the constant fear that somehow the various insurance programs of which I was part would figure out a way to exclude me because of my preexisting condition. From day to day I tried not to think about how frequently and urgently I required these injections. Later in life, I made an estimate of how many times I had had to strap on a tourniquet, clean my skin with alcohol, and push a needle through my own skin and into my vein. It came to over ten thousand times.

*

After years of being the stranger—disabled in elementary school, a foreigner in high school—I mostly wanted to fit in, and I was delighted that I made friends so quickly. Given my enthusiasm at the time for everything about Princeton, I am not so surprised, looking back, that I was pleased to be approached in my sophomore year about joining the most exclusive club on campus, known as Ivy Club.

The "eating clubs" are a Princeton oddity that arose during the nineteenth century. They were, in essence, fraternities that admitted juniors and seniors. Each eating club had its own elegant and spacious headquarters on Prospect Street near campus. Each sported a dining room, library, game room, and backyard. A few of them even had ballrooms, into which they imported bands, women from other colleges, and large amounts of liquor on weekends. They were the huge party engines that drove campus social life all year long.

I had heard about the clubs when I was applying to Princeton, and I was concerned that they might be strongholds of division and snobbery. No, no, no! I was told by the admissions office and by the students with whom I met during campus visits. They were simply places that served three meals a day, provided a quiet place to study, and held parties. Besides, I was told, they weren't even really part of the university. They were independent associations, run by their own boards and maintained by their own endowments.

By the time I arrived there, the university had three kinds of clubs: selective clubs that only admitted men, selective clubs that admitted men and women, and "open" clubs, which admitted anyone who signed up. The university provided food and recreational facilities for freshmen and sophomores, but it did not have the capacity to cover all the students on campus, which meant that it was depending on the clubs to provide a key university service.

The annual selection process went by the weird name of "bicker." The decision of whether to participate came to most students in the fall of their sophomore year. Club members recruited younger students to become part of the process, and the students in turn sidled up to members to express their interest. I was astonished when several members of Ivy Club started dropping by my room or seeking me out in the hulking dining halls around campus. *We would like you to see what it is like*, they said. *Will you come for dinner tomorrow night?*

Sure, I replied.

My closest friends grimaced at me. I had already developed a reputation as someone with passionate views, sometimes conservative, more often progressive. How could I be willing to explore membership in a club—in *Ivy*, of all places?

I listened and I thought, Well, maybe they are right. But it couldn't hurt to take a look.

I visited Ivy and I was bowled over. It was physically beautiful, with an elegant entry, a comfortable and well-designed living room, a billiards room, and a magnificent wood-paneled dining room. The "men of Ivy" sat at a single long table, where they were served meals prepared by a large kitchen staff and served by waiters in tuxedos and white gloves. They ate off china and silver. When I went upstairs to the library, I found a stylish chamber with oriental rugs, a roaring fire, and endless rows of leather-bound books. Sitting in one of the comfy reading chairs at the end of the room, I noticed a set of elegant books within hand's reach. They were rare copies of Woodrow Wilson's five-volume masterwork, *A History of the American People*, written while he was a professor at Princeton and before he became the president of Princeton, the governor of New Jersey, and the president of the United States. I idly pulled one volume off the shelf and opened it to the first page. To my surprise, I found Wilson's autograph. In fact, he had signed all five.

Yes, the place was lovely in a conservative, English way, and yes, the food was excellent, but that is not what drew me in. It was something more alluring. I had grown up without brothers, I had never seriously participated in an athletic team, and I had not been able to join the military, so I had no experience of extended male camaraderie. And here were these charming, relaxed, and friendly young men, all of them ready with a funny quip or a helpful hand, inviting me to become one of their band. It touched an inner desire that had lingered within me for years. I went through the long interview process during the first week of February 1976.

Late one night at the end of the week I found that an envelope had been slipped under my door in the dormitory. My heart jumped. The expensive stationery bore the symbol of an ivy leaf.

I was in.

*

My daily participation at Ivy did not begin until the following fall. I endured the silly initiation rite and enjoyed the banter over every meal. I learned to play billiards. I went to parties where I drank too much, an experience that taught me that however good the alcohol buzz might feel in the short term, it wasn't worth the misery of throwing up all night in a toilet stall. I made excellent use of the library; every night after dinner I would go up there, lay out my books, and work in silence with the fire crackling behind me for four hours. My grades skyrocketed.

As the weather turned cool and the novelty wore off, I noticed some unexpected aspects of the club's life. The nervous sophomores who had entered with me the previous spring had now turned into solid juniors who would soon be leading the club. They asked me to start recruiting the next class. What sort of person were they looking for? I asked. They gave me a garbled answer. They wanted someone who was unusual, who was a leader, who stood out, who added spice to the mix. And also someone who was likable, a regular guy, a team player, who would fit in. They scanned the directory of sophomores to pick out famous names. They brought a string of perfectly friendly but bland roommates and teammates to dinner, trying to make the case that they would be perfect.

Slowly I saw my surroundings in a new light. How had I gotten in? I wondered. Perhaps I fell into the celebrity category, since my parents were well-known writers who had published a book about how our family coped with hemophilia. I had been on game shows and national news as part of the publicity for that book. I noticed abruptly that the great majority of the cooking staff and the silent waiters were black, while the huge majority of club members were white. Sometimes when I emerged from the front door of Ivy to return to campus, I crossed paths with African-American and Latino and Asian students who were on their way to the Third World Center, a kind of open club for students of color. In a detail that seemed particularly insensitive on the university administration's part, these students had to walk every day up and down a long street, past every one of the clubs, with their glowing yellow windows and burbling music, before they reached their gathering place. The clubs did not have a formal policy of excluding minority students, and every club had a few hardy members who were willing to put up with being virtually alone among their peers. Still, the cultural and class divide was communicated clearly through their styles. Ivy radiated English Men's Club. Cap and Gown was Great Gatsby. Tiger Club was Animal House. Even Terrace, which was an open club, became famous for its throwback hippie tone, serving endless trays of roasted veg-etables and half-cooked eggplant smothered in giant gobs of melted Muenster cheese.

As I went back and forth to my dorm room, I wrestled with a new set of dilemmas about inclusion and exclusion. Yes, I was in, but a lot of people, people I respected, were out. And while Princeton spent a lot of time using its admission and scholar-ship policies to assemble a diverse student body, why did it then make sense to resegregate the students for their last two years? They were making individual decisions about whether and what to join, but wasn't it a system that rewarded and molded those who were accepted by this social sorting system and silenced those who were not? I was having a wonderful time with this new group of male friends, but did my enjoy-ment depend on excluding the women in my class whom I had come to know, to admire, and in some cases to love?

What troubled me more than anything was the slow hard-ening of my club friends' attitudes toward the realities and principles at stake. Those who benefited from the system slowly and imperceptibly began to justify it. Those who had chosen not to participate dismissed it. Those who had been rejected resented it. To my dismay, I felt that I was witnessing the intensification of the very kind of discrimination and mis-understanding that I had observed and rejected in my experi-ences with race, with disabilities, and with human rights.

The ironies abounded. I was a student at a highly selective university that used exclusion to create a theoretically inclu-sive community. And then, to escape the anonymity of crowds and the unwelcome burden (to the administration) of providing for everyone, we broke up that same inclusive community with a new form of intensified exclusion.

It was disturbing. No, it was more than disturbing, I decided. It was wrong.

So the question became what to do—not just about myself and my own participation, but about the system as a whole. With this challenge I tackled for the first time the vexing question of strategy. It was not enough to have an intuitive sense of injustice. I realized that I needed to select a goal and then design the process to achieve it. But I had no idea how to do this.

I started with what I knew best, the impulsive act. I knew I had to quit Ivy. This time, however, I pondered the time and place in advance. At first I decided to go all the way through Bicker Week to select the next class and then quietly resign a few weeks later. As we began interviewing candidates, however, the arbitrary nature of our process became more and more evident. Every visiting candidate had an index card on which the interviewers recorded their impressions and indicated their preference: an up arrow for admission, a down arrow for rejection, and a sideways arrow for indifference. To signal my growing objections, I gave every person I talked to an up arrow, until my actions were detected by the club president, who took me aside to scold me. I kept doing it anyway.

The actual process of selection took place over two all-night meetings in the first week of the second term. The aura of secrecy and the bodily trial of sleeplessness had the effect of binding the club members even more tightly together. I realized that if I quit before the first night, I would never know what it was really like—and I would probably be accused of being too weak physically to endure the challenge. So I diligently sat through the first marathon. As the night wore on and exhaustion set in, the standards of admission and the conversations that surrounded them became more and more peculiar. The group focused on each candidate in turn, and when the discussion opened up, it became a swirling mix of impressions, hearsay, personal details, team affiliations, lasting grudges, and primitive psychoanalysis. I looked around at my friends—for they still were my friends—and felt deeply unhappy, for them and for myself.

The next night we retired to the library again after dinner and attacked the remainder of the list. We spent more than two and a half hours on one poor fellow who had staked his college life and reputation on admission to the club. One of his closest friends finally sank him by saying that his fascination with Ivy was the sign of a weak and dependent character. At the end of the discussion, he was voted down. (I later learned that he sank into such misery that he transferred to another college.)

I had arbitrarily selected midnight as the moment of my announcement. I waited until we had completed voting on the person at hand, and then I stood up.

"I have something to say," I said to the group.

They looked at me, tired, curious, uncertain.

"I was proud to be admitted to this club," I began. "I have enjoyed my time here. I like you all very much. Some of you have been especially good friends to me." I scanned their faces and choked up slightly. Perhaps I was making a terrible mistake?

"At the same time I think we are part of a system that is unfair and unjust. I don't agree with excluding women. And I don't believe we have the right to sit in judgment like this over our friends and classmates from the same college. Our friendship within the club should not be purchased at the price of their rejection."

They were silent, and I could sense an undercurrent of anger.

"I feel no alternative but to resign. Which I am doing immediately. Thank you. And goodbye."

I walked out of the room, through the carpeted halls, down the carved staircase, and out the front door. My little electric cart was parked in front, in the snow. I turned it on and headed down the dark street toward my room. I was breathing hard, struggling with my emotions. As I drove away, I looked up at the sky and saw the moon hanging implacably in the ice-cold air. For a moment I was distracted by its brilliance, and by the cool magnanimity—or indifference—of its presence in the sky.

When I looked down again, I realized that I had done something irrevocable.

I was now out.

*

The weeks that followed offered a healthy lesson in the emotions stirred up by change. My regular circle of friends—those who had never joined clubs—patted me on the back and teased me because it had taken me too long. My girlfriend smiled at me. I swiftly received several phone calls from club members saying that they supported my actions and admired me. *Great, I said, then let's discuss how the club could be reformed. Maybe the club could start by admitting women. Did you want to meet and talk about this? Absolutely,* they said in cautious tones. *Let's do that. In a few weeks.*

Others let it be known that my actions confirmed their long-time suspicions that I was a self-righteous jerk. A few did indeed dredge up the medical argument: I was said to have "collapsed" in the meeting. Perhaps the most surprising complaint—which over the years that followed I often heard in response to actions that pushed for change—was that I was right in *principle*, but I had blown the *timing*. Wasn't I aware that there were confidential discussions about changing the club's rules? It had been going so well, until I acted foolishly. Now, sadly, the opportunity for change had passed. My actions had backfired and I had no one to blame but myself.

I did have one meeting with about a dozen friends, who represented nearly a third of the club's junior class members. I was excited. This was nearly a majority, and the people in the room would be in positions of power the next year. We mapped out some possible steps. Tentative agreements were reached. I emerged hopeful about the future.

This effort quickly ran out of gas. Though I was disappointed, I understood what had happened. My friends, many of whom I still respected, decided that this was some weird preoccupation of mine. The system really wasn't that bad.

There was no need to speak; I was no longer a thorn in their side; out of sight, out of mind; silence is acquiescence.

I went through the spring and summer pondering what to do. I analyzed the calendar strategically. Bicker survived each year because the actual choosing came up suddenly in the dead of winter. The choices and consequences were so swift that there was little time to react. Within a few months the seniors graduated and the juniors took control, and the whole dance continued.

This time, however, we would start organizing early, in September. With a group of friends I created the "Social Alternatives Coalition." Our goal was to push the clubs to open up and the university to create a college system, including a student center, which, incredibly, we did not have. Dozens of people came to our weekly meetings, and we followed a very loose form of democratic decision-making in which anyone who was in the room could vote. This meant that one week one group of students would decide one thing, and the next week a different cast of characters would decide something else. I chaired the meetings, torn between my delight at the growing engagement and frustrated by the uneven and unpredictable process. Eventually we lurched into a major decision: we were going to hold a demonstration on Prospect Street during Bicker Week.

Suddenly I was the head of an organizing campaign. To get our message out without money for flyers (the Internet, of course, did not yet exist), we simply decided to call every student in the school. We tore the school phone directory into columns and handed them out to dozens of volunteers. This worked well: rooms with more than one occupant got more than one call. Every club member was informed of what was going to happen. We arranged for candles and bullhorns and all the other paraphernalia of public marches. We notified the administration and the local police.

When the day came, I went over to Prospect Street an hour early with two or three fellow organizers. It was winter again, and the sky was cold and gray. For a long time we waited, and no one showed up. Well, that's okay, I thought. I will walk up and back with this small band and then I can retreat into my humiliation. At least it will be over.

And then people arrived, dozens and dozens and dozens. Eventually more than four hundred people gathered in front of the Woodrow Wilson School. We began our march, shuffling quietly along the sidewalk with our candles. There were a few signs, and occasionally people broke into chants, but mostly the march was solemn. When I passed Ivy Club, I glanced over and thought I saw a few faces looking through the curtains. I sighed with sorrow, wondering if I could have done something else to persuade my friends.

The next day the student paper announced that we had held the largest demonstration since the Vietnam War. The president of the university immediately appointed two committees. The first, the Committee on Undergraduate Residential Life, or CURL, was made up of students, faculty, and administrators. The second was made up of trustees who were designated to receive and debate the CURL report when it came through.

One assistant dean came up to me in the months that followed and said that the administrators had been looking for some ways to make changes, but they could not initiate them for fear of the reaction of the alumni and trustees who were still angry about admitting women. Our march had provided the impetus to act.

And oddly enough, it all worked. A participant in the march, Sally Frank, filed a lawsuit against one of the male clubs for banning her from admission. The clubs argued that they were private establishments, independent of the university. Sally, who advanced the case during her remaining years in college, in law school, and then as a law professor, argued that the university and the clubs were inextricably bound. There were no members who were not students. The university relied on the clubs to provide services it could not offer. Thus the clubs should be held accountable under the same rules barring discrimination among public accommodations. The case cranked on for fourteen years, until it reached the New Jersey Supreme Court. The court agreed with Frank and ordered the all-male clubs to admit women.

The CURL process also took decades and continued through three university presidents. Eventually the committee issued a report calling for Princeton to institute a college system. The trustees accepted it, and the university raised hundreds of millions of dollars to pay for these new internal entities.

Today Princeton has six residential colleges. Some of the clubs remain selective, but all admit women. It took nearly thirty years, but through the hard work of hundreds of people, it is a less discriminatory campus.

"Do you think thirty years is a long time or a short time for major institutional change?" I asked a classmate over dinner about a year ago.

He paused and thought for a moment. "Of course in some ways it should have happened much faster," he said. "But then again, there is always the chance that it might never have happened at all."

CHAPTER FIVE

Faith AND *Fortune*

When was it that we saw you a stranger and welcomed
you, or naked and gave you clothing? And when was it
that we saw you sick or in prison and visited you?

MATTHEW 25: 38−39

While we were still in France, we visited the great cathedrals and monasteries—Notre Dame, Beauvais, Sainte-Chapelle, Mont Saint Michel—and each time I found myself deeply moved. The soaring stone, the stunning stained glass windows, and the cool, peaceful interiors flickering with thousands of candles quelled me into silence whenever I stepped inside. On the site of the magnificent cathedral of Chartres, fifty miles outside Paris, five churches had risen in sequence before the final building began to take shape nearly a thousand years ago. The idea that more than fifty generations of men and women had devoted themselves to the building, protection, and improvement of this place of worship astonished me.

I had grown up as a nominal Christian; our family attended

church at Christmas and Easter and a few other times a year. I had enjoyed my engagement with a church youth group in Paris, but I did not feel I understood the world's religions, or my own supposed faith. I wanted to remedy this, so over the years I occasionally dipped into the Bible, particularly the four gospels of Matthew, Mark, Luke, and John, trying to read these unusual stories for myself.

I discovered, to my surprise, that most of my early impressions about Jesus of Nazareth had been false. Throughout my childhood Jesus had appeared to me as a benevolent authority figure, friendly in an abstract way, a distant leader venerated in stone and stained glass and in the tedious words of centuries-old prayers. As a teenager I thought that the whole enterprise of church reeked of hypocrisy, which in my calculus was perhaps the greatest of all sins. Through my youthful eyes the world was a mess, and much of the responsibility lay with the unwillingness of religious people to live up to the beautiful and challenging words of their own faiths.

To my surprise, I learned when I opened up the New Testament that Jesus had agreed with this critique. Instead of appearing as a kind of super-parent, handing out exhortations to people who were bad to be good, Jesus reserved his most acute, and in some cases blistering, criticism for those who took on the trappings and practice of religion but then used their piety as an excuse to judge and condemn others. He explicitly confronted those who were preoccupied with superficial forms of public behavior while they neglected the deeper demand for justice, for love, for humility, and for reconciliation.

In the texts Jesus comes across as a lively, dynamic, restlessly compassionate man. He chooses not to distribute approval to the pious, and he offers encouragement to people struggling with faith. "Go and learn what this means," he says at one point. " 'I desire mercy and not sacrifice.' " He attacks the professionally religious for obeying small rules of behavior and missing the core purpose of a life of faith. "Woe to you scribes and Pharisees, hypocrites," he says in the Gospel of Matthew, "for . . . you have neglected the more important matters of the law, like justice and mercy and faithfulness."

This unexpected splash of cold water woke me up. During one summer while I was still in high school, I suffered a bleeding that left me immobilized for a week. Looking for something to read, I picked up the Bible and worked my way through the gospels. Again I was struck by Jesus' energy, his restlessness, his bubbling passion. And having learned that about him, I was less surprised to read that he regularly felt great frustration when his message did not seem to penetrate the minds of those who loved him and followed him closely. To many he said sadly, "You have eyes but you do not see, you have ears but you do not hear." And in one of the most poignant passages of all, he evoked the image of children using music to try to elicit some kind of response, happy or sad, and failing, implicitly likening this to his own inability to generate a response:

To what shall I compare this present generation?
　You are like children calling to each other in the
marketplace,

"I piped for you and you would not dance;
I wailed for you and you would not mourn."

This person, whose two-thousand-year-old story was sitting in millions of bookshelves and pews, was not, by my reading, someone who floated with gentle detachment above the sufferings of the world. This was a man who loved those around him with an intensity that even he sometimes found hard to bear.

My own faith was still in its early stages, but what I read moved me and drew me in. I didn't know if I really understood it, or if I could live up to it, but the reverberations of his fervent way of seeing the world began to resonate inside me. And once that resonance started, it started me down a path of wonderment and growth and change.

*

While I was in college, I considered becoming a minister, but I rejected the idea decisively. It seemed like the ministry would demand too high a standard of behavior. I knew my own weaknesses and flaws, and I knew that even if I managed to control my greed, resentment, pettiness, lust, and pride, they would all still reside within me—and somehow that seemed even worse than acting on them. How could I pretend to be someone pure and loving when there were plenty of moments when I was not? How could I represent an institution with so many glorious ideals and so many ugly historical failures? The answer seemed clear: I could not.

The decisive moment came for me at the end of my years in college, when I experienced a reawakening of my faith that is difficult to describe and even more difficult to explain. It came at a time when I felt broken and adrift, uncertain about my deepest values and my direction. I was not sure whether God existed and whether it mattered. I felt caught in a spiral of expectations about what I desired to be and knowledge of how frequently I failed. And at that point I met a young woman who asked me a very simple question: Had I ever mentioned my unhappiness in prayer? Had I ever actually spoken to God about the matter?

I was embarrassed to say no. My first reaction was that it didn't make sense to do so. Later I turned the thought around: What could I lose if I tried it? The greatest risk, it seemed to me, would be silence—and the resulting disappointment. So outside on a small bench one evening I cast my prayer into the vastness of the world, as one might throw a message in a bottle into the sea. My prayer rambled, but it was heartfelt.

I don't seem to have done the best with my life. I am not on the path to becoming the person I want to be—someone who is gracious and courageous, loving and trustworthy. I am not that good at caring about others. I don't know how to move forward. And I would like to know if you exist. Jesus, if you are out there, I would like you to be part of my life.

And oddly enough, that's all it took. I didn't see lights and I didn't hear voices, but when I opened my eyes I felt different.

Profoundly different. A burden had been lifted from my heart. I could breathe. The part of me that had felt empty since my birth felt complete. And, more than anything, I felt awash in grace.

We all go through life carrying so much guilt and anxiety; we are constantly being measured and judged. In many of our daily roles we are expected to meet ever higher standards: as students and employees, as children and parents. We are told that our identity and our success depend on our performance, and we have internalized this message all the way into our deepest core. But the message of God's grace—the center of the "good news" proclaimed by Jesus—is that in the eyes of the one who really matters, the Being who gave us our being, our performance is immaterial. We are endlessly, boundlessly loved. This love is not a sentimental characteristic that over-looks the innumerable ways in which human beings have hurt themselves and each other or that ignores the self-centered qualities in all of our lives. I came to believe that God is fully conscious of these, yet fully forgiving. Love is not an emotion and it does not hinge on behavior: it is an irrevocable decision about the essence of humanity and about each person, made by God in advance, which stands as a counterbalance and a cure to our endless self-judgment and fear.

When I experienced this reawakening of my faith, just before the fall of my senior year in college, I wanted to under-stand how people in previous centuries and in our own had responded to this kind of experience. Returning to campus, I discovered that there were not many people to talk to about this, and so I did what many of my peers were doing when they wanted deeper exposure to a topic: I enrolled in graduate school. I received a scholarship from Yale Divinity School, a program that seemed to combine the intellectual rigor I wanted with the humanity and warmth that would make the exploration worthwhile.

I arrived in the fall of 1978, and I swept through some of the happiest weeks of my life. I instantly fell in with new friends who treated each other differently from any group of people I had ever met. They were warm, thoughtful, attentive, curious, and unusually happy. Most, but not all, of them were Christians of one denomination or another. Some were recent graduates, like me, and others were coming back to school to pursue ministry as a second career. There were many women, some of whom had to show real grit in applying for positions of leadership in churches that still resisted the idea of women's ordination. I was a throwback to an older model of ministry student: I was a young man who had come directly from college.

I spent the crisp fall evenings throwing Frisbees on the green or playing my guitar in the dorm. I bought a huge stack of books with tiny print that I carried back and forth to the library. I made friends not only among the students but also among the faculty. One of my closest friends was a Catholic priest named Henri Nouwen, who I later learned was one of America's most popular spiritual authors at the time. I often visited Henri's daily services of communion to enter a deep place of reflection and peace.

Even as I experienced the warmth of this exceptional community, I was not sure that I was going to pursue an actual career in the ministry. Still, everything proceeded wonderfully well for the first ten weeks, until just before Thanksgiving, when I came down with an illness that no one could identify. The symptoms resembled the flu, and I suffered from moments of extreme lethargy, when I could barely move or make decisions. I reported this to my doctors in New York, who urged me to go to Yale–New Haven Hospital in case I was experiencing a cerebral hemorrhage.

For five days the doctors performed tests. Was it the flu? Or some other virus? Or perhaps even a seizure disorder? They scanned my body and analyzed my brain waves, but they came up with nothing. Although my condition improved, I lost the energy to do all the things that my schedule required. I muscled through the next few weeks to finish my exams, but when I returned after Christmas, I realized that the unnamed condition was still plaguing me. With enormous regret I said goodbye to my friends, withdrew from school, and went home.

It was not easy living again with my parents, in my childhood room, without knowing what was bothering me or what I would do next. My friends were all making great strides in school or in their first jobs, while I was adrift. Slowly my physical condition improved, but I was still without direction and purpose.

*

After a long car trip exploring the United States, I moved to Washington, D.C. I was fortunate to get a job as a researcher for Congress Watch, an organization that focused on the hidden pathways of dollars and influence that affected decisions in Congress. I worked directly for Mark Green, a dynamic young lawyer who had already written half a dozen books as part of Ralph Nader's network. Nader at that time was still doing extraordinary work on behalf of American consumers, and he had set up small advocacy groups that focused on different topics, such as pharmaceuticals and health-care reform, automobile and transportation policy, and corruption in Congress. Though I later broke with him over his decision to run for president in both 2000 and 2004, in the 1980s I found him a provocative and in many cases inspired analyst of the structure of the American economy and the flaws in our politics. Mark Green was an equally brilliant scholar and organizer and went on to be elected president of the New York City Council (known as the "public advocate") and to run as a candidate for both the U.S. Senate and the mayoralty of New York City.

When I arrived in Washington, Jimmy Carter had been president for three years, and he was gearing up for his reelection campaign in 1980. I immediately fell in with a dynamic network from different parts of the American activist community: environmentalists, labor leaders, consumer advocates, and elected officials. The Republican Party and the corporate interests that tended to support it had been pushed back forcefully after the Watergate scandal, leading to the election of a huge number of new congressional representatives in 1974 and the election of Carter in 1976.

By late 1979 the political mood of the country was changing. The inflation and unemployment rates were running unacceptably high. In November 1979, radical students invaded the U.S. embassy in Teheran and took fifty-two embassy employees hostage, triggering a year-long standoff. Carter, anticipating conservative pressure, seemed to many of us to be trimming his sails and slowing down on his commitments to progressive causes. Still, it seemed unlikely that the nation was about to take a major turn to the right. To many, Ronald Reagan seemed unelectable in early 1980 because of his strong brand of conservatism and because he was sixty-nine years old. Our job that year was to remind the president that he needed to stay faithful to the coalition that had elected him.

We also wanted to educate voters around the country about corporate power. I was initially given the responsibility of investigating the role of large corporations abroad—something I was naturally interested in because of South Africa—but increasingly my assignments focused on the behavior of a few large U.S. corporations and the role of aggressive business lobbying organizations, such as the National Association of Manufacturers and the U.S. Chamber of Commerce.

Eventually I became the national research director for a network of organizations that were behind what became known as "Big Business Day." Modeled loosely on Earth Day, which had been established ten years before and in which many of my new associates had been involved, the idea was to hold teach-ins and demonstrations around the country to object to the increasingly aggressive influence of corporations on government at all levels. Though not all corporations took such a belligerent approach, we were seeing a surge in corporate campaign money entering politics, attacks on environmental regulations, soaring executive pay, slashed hourly wages, attempts to dismantle workers' rights and labor unions, and fierce battles over consumer and product safety standards for everything from drugs to toys to automobiles. We also saw a refusal to consider energy efficiency and unquestioning support for right-wing regimes (like that in South Africa), where business felt it had a freer hand. Our effort was not simply a list of complaints but a campaign to provoke a deeper discussion about the relationship between economic power and democracy.

Around Thanksgiving in 1979 I received a phone call from Ralph Nader himself, asking me to take on a particularly challenging task. Would I create an anthology of articles on corporations in America? Sure, I responded—when did he need it? Well, he said, it needed to be published the week before Big Business Day in April.

"What?" I said. "That's only four months from now! How can we gather, select, compile, edit, and print an anthology from scratch in four months?"

"I'm sure you can do it," he replied.

This was a much bigger task at that time than it would be today. There were no personal computers and no such thing as word processing. There was no Internet, no Google, and no e-mail. Everything would have to be done by hand. I immediately went to the Library of Congress, which had just invented a new cataloguing system that included a large number of recently published books and articles. One could gain access to the library's ancient computer terminals only by waiting in a long line, and then one was limited to two hours at a time.

For the next few weeks I lived there, entering a vast list of key words about corporate responsibility and printing out piles of sheets that had the waxy texture of early faxes. When my time ran out, I simply got back in line and waited until my turn came up again. While I stood in line, I checked off the articles that looked interesting, and every night I edited the list down to those that seemed the most promising. Fortunately I was able to attract a small army of volunteers, who fanned out across the library to make photocopies of the articles that might be included in the anthology. Every evening, working late into the night, I read the articles and assigned scores to them, looking at the appropriateness of the topic and the quality of the writing.

Within a month I had just over a hundred possible articles for the anthology, and a month after that I had boiled the list down to fifty-two. By the end of March the book was ready for publication by Pilgrim Press, and it came out the week of Big Business Day, with Mark Green and me as coeditors. Organized under broad headings such as "The Corporation and Health," "The Corporation and Natural Resources," "The Impact of Multinationals," and "Corporate Governance," the book had strong, detailed entries on agribusiness, pharmaceuticals, chemicals, mining, oil, and automobiles. We looked at controversies over toxic sites, asbestos, union busting, industry advertising in classrooms, plant relocation, corporate lobbying, and campaign donations. We chronicled specific battles being fought over unionization in southern textile plants, the marketing of Nestlé infant formula, the shipping of hazardous waste to third world countries, international consumerism, and investment in South Africa. We probed problems in the field of energy, including the dominance of fossil fuels, the distribution of ownership rights within solar power, and the risks of nuclear plants. We evaluated approaches that had been proposed or were being debated about the correct relationship among government, regulation, innovation, economic prosperity, and the protection of public rights. There were also thoughtful articles by major authors on how corporations are structured and managed, about board interlocks, mergers and acquisitions, executive compensation, market concentration, and political involvement.

All in all, two things strike me, looking at the list thirty years later. The first is that the issues raised were comprehensive, important, and in many cases urgent. The other is that after three decades, many of these issues are still being fought—and in some cases, after twenty years of Republican presidents and aggressive lobbying by business associations, the circumstances have become worse. In 1980 it was still possible to imagine the United States Congress proposing, debating, and perhaps even passing a "Corporate Democracy Act," which would have required a majority of board members to be independent, asked boards to oversee particular areas of corporate management (including audit and legal compliance), and prohibited board interlocks with other corporations. It was a bold move that, had it been enacted even in part, might have forestalled the financial manipulation and the distortions in corporate governance that damaged the economy over the following twenty years.

Today many of the problems have grown greater, and have led to protests in the streets all over the world, including the United States. Corporate power continues to rise, bringing with it enormous changes and influence. The willingness to imagine new forms of accountability and new pathways to prosperity has, in the public realm, sadly shrunk. In the early part of this century, discussions about the next phase of capitalism and the redesign of the American economy have only just started.

*

Though the timing of my year in Washington was precipitated by my mysterious illness, I had always intended to step back from divinity school for a while to consider my vocation. In most Christian denominations one must pursue two parallel tracks to being ordained to the ministry. The first track is within the church organization itself—one has to run a gauntlet of interviews, approvals, commissions, psychological tests, meetings with bishops or other church authorities, and chaplaincy training, all of which are designed to explore the underlying motivations and skills of the person who wants to be ordained. Though complex, these requirements make sense, because ordination authorizes a minister to speak not only on behalf of a specific church but for the denomination and even the whole faith. Because persons in congregations invest enormous trust in their pastors, the people chosen for those positions of leadership must prove worthy of that trust.

The second track is the acquisition of a master's degree from an accredited program. The Episcopal Church required steady progress on both tracks within a defined amount of time. I had to attend all the meetings and interviews set up by the denomination, concluding with one or more meetings with the diocesan bishop, who had the final say.

After my year in Washington I realized that I was more committed to community leadership than ever, that I was growing in my faith, and that I was not just ready but eager to continue on the path. At the same time, I had been plunged more and more deeply into the world of business and economics. The topics I had studied in college and during my year in Washington went to the heart of the challenge of how a person should articulate and remain faithful to his or her core principles in the hustle and bustle of modern economic life.

When I arrived back on the Yale Divinity School campus, my mind was buzzing with questions, ranging from the tightly practical to the broadly theoretical, many of them focused on economic theory and American business. I had seen from many angles that American business was an enormous engine of change—the most potent force in our century. Its impact on society rivaled or exceeded the influence of ancient kings, or the huge control exercised by the Roman Catholic Church in Europe for many centuries.

The modern corporation had grown organically. The earliest corporate charters had been granted by the king, or by the government, for a limited period of time and with a specific public purpose in mind. A tiny number of corporations, such as the Dutch East India Company, became early multinationals, dispatching their vessels to all the corners of the earth, controlling large markets, and in some places, such as seventeenth-century America and South Africa, even hiring captains and ships to establish permanent outposts on distant shores. Both New York City and Cape Town were settled by expeditions authorized by European kings yet paid for by the Dutch East India Company.

Because the modern corporation is relatively new, it never occurred to early political theorists to wonder what would happen if this particular form of human organization became so wealthy and powerful that it might rival governments for power. In the formation of the United States, the founders worried about many different forms of human aggregation that might cause trouble for the fledgling democracy, and they worried the most about "factions." We can only speculate how they would have factored in the political power of mammoth corporations, some of which now control unimaginable riches, globe-spanning assets, and armies of employees. There are ample reasons to suspect that they would have had reservations about the legal fiction and political status of corporate "personhood," because these "persons," unlike humans, are both immortal and amoral.

Everywhere I looked, I saw the effects, talents, and influence of business. Businesses took all forms, from the local corner store where I bought milk to the multinational behemoths that could reshape almost any place on earth. The bigger they became, the more breathtaking their capacity was; the largest firms, acting with broad legal rights and sometimes without legal constraints, could gather and apply hundreds of millions of dollars to any project of their choosing. In some ways they were amazingly effective: they had the capability to organize human cooperation across cities, states, and nations; they had figured out how to combine vastly different skills to attain a single objective; and they could identify specific goals and then implement all the steps necessary to achieve them.

At the same time, some corporations took steps that were impossible to align with even the most elementary standards of human morality. Any action—and every action—seemed to be justified as long as someone somewhere could concoct an argument (no matter how tenuous) that it would be beneficial to the shareholders. Investing in destructive products or industries; trading with dictators on both left and right; corrupting democratic institutions and processes; manipulating markets toward monopoly; engaging in price-fixing, kickbacks, excessive pay, intimidation, firings, union-busting, and layoffs; distributing inadequately tested products and chemicals for business and consumer use; destroying forests, oceans, waterways, open land; devastating communities after plant closings—all of these things were justified by the supposedly self-correcting virtue of the free market and portrayed as necessary to human prosperity.

I found the combination of business and politics particularly toxic. Politics, though a messy and imperfect field, was tasked—at least in theory—with the objectives of protecting and pursuing the common good. Many businesses agreed with this goal and asked only that they not be so smothered in regulation that they would be prevented from creating the jobs and investing in the products of the future. But other companies had very different objectives and much more aggressive tactics. They employed huge numbers of lobbyists to bend legislation to their advantage, either by inserting special benefits or by ripping out provisions that they didn't like. They maintained stables of lawyers, both inside and outside the firm, ready to attack anyone who seemed like a threat. And some of them spent considerable money on political donations to make sure that their voices would be heard at critical—and often secret—moments.

*

I arrived back at Yale Divinity School filled with new information and questions about wealth and poverty, cooperation and competition, political and economic justice, fairness and efficiency, and I wondered what my newfound field of theology and ethics might have to say about them. I had been exposed to the fascinating power of the modern corporation, and I believed that these entities raised complicated and important questions about the kind of world we want to live in. I looked forward to taking a few courses on the relationship between economics and ethics, or politics and social justice, or money and morality.

To my dismay, I discovered that there weren't any. Not only

that, there were few people who knew enough about them to offer a perspective. I had a wonderful faculty, deeply schooled in the historical controversies of past eras. I could learn about the early church fathers' attitudes toward the accumulation of wealth, about Martin Luther's essays on usury, or about the role of religion in the perpetuation and then the abolition of slavery. There was even the occasional lecture on economic development in Third World countries or in inner cities, or about specific controversies like human rights or the sale of infant formula in underdeveloped nations. If I was looking for a clear, thoughtful review of America's economy and of the functioning of the modern corporation, with special attention to how people of communities of faith or specific local churches should approach them, there was nothing.

Equally surprising to me was that the institution that I was coming to know and understand well—the church—was also largely silent on many issues central to daily life. To my mind, many churches were often slow to identify new questions or injustice that might challenge long-held assumptions. Part of the problem was the result of the periodic swing back and forth between two visions of ministry, the prophetic and the pastoral. A prophetic ministry focuses on speaking about the world, pointing out the gap between reality and aspiration, and urging change. A pastoral ministry put the emphasis on personal interactions between people of faith, in which individuals encourage and support each other. I discovered while I was in divinity school that the pendulum of education had swung strongly toward the pastoral. The structural critique that had flourished throughout the 1960s was steadily being replaced in the 1980s by a focus on the needs of individuals and families. Though I understood and supported my many friends who devoted themselves to this role, I remained perplexed that one of the most important institutions in modern society—the business firm—was never covered in class, discussed over meals, or preached from the pulpit. It was as though certain structures in society had grown so prevalent and powerful that they became invisible. This was a mystery to me. Was it possible that one could be so close to something that one could no longer see it?

This peculiar invisibility may have reflected an age-old debate within Christianity about whether Christians should consider themselves active parts of this world, in all its complexity and contradiction, or adhere to a set of values that were by definition radically different. Put another way, in what way should one's beliefs alter one's behavior? Even John the Baptist had been asked by a cross-sampling of his followers what they should actually do to put his message of repentance into daily practice. And Jesus had been understood by some of his followers to say that Christians should allow their daily and most conventional actions to be guided by faith in God while suggesting that the world was governed by false assumptions and would soon be replaced.

Another possible explanation why people in seminaries did not talk about economic life is that they simply did not know much about it. How many divinity school students—or faculty—got up every morning filled with curiosity about what was going to be on the business page? How many divinity school students had a background in business or training in finance or management? When I was in school, the answer was very few. I immediately tried to increase the number of opportunities for the divinity school community to learn more about the corporate world. I organized a small discussion group called the Economics and Ethics Research Center and even won a few small research grants to look at specific problems in Connecticut. I designed a course on corporate responsibility and somehow persuaded two faculty members to teach it with me.

Faced with my intense interest, people sometimes marveled or objected. "But how can you talk about all these things when you don't really know anything about business?" In one sense it was an attack on my credentials, and thus my right to speak. I have always rejected this point of view as undemocratic. Citizens should be able to discuss anything they want and apply whatever values seem relevant to them. If we start barring people from conversations because they lack professional training, our ability to talk about our collective choices will erode.

At the same time, I recognized that there was an element of truth in my fellow students' criticism. Despite my reading, my course, and my time in Washington, there were still many things I did not understand about business. If my intention was to become a strong and fair advocate for integrating economic creativity and political or religious purpose, then I needed to learn more. Within a year of returning to divinity school, I had applied for and was admitted to a two-year degree program at the Yale School of Management, which was to begin the following year.

At this time I was also under the supervision of the Episcopal bishop of New York, Paul Moore, Jr. Paul was the model of a patrician clergyman, born on an enormous estate in Long Island and educated at St. Paul's and Yale. He had become an officer in the Marines and was wounded in battle. When he returned to civilian life, he could easily have become an investment banker or a politician. But he chose the ministry and launched on a bold career as a leader for social justice, taking positions in poor churches, leading marches, and speaking out fearlessly. He led the national church forward on civil rights and was one of the first bishops to ordain women. Given his breeding and appearance—he was as tall as a flagpole, with silver hair and a gravelly bass voice—it was perhaps inevitable that he would become a bishop. Eventually he became bishop of New York, presiding over the largest diocese and the largest cathedral in the country, St. John the Divine. Because I was within his jurisdiction, I had been sent to him. He would make the ultimate decision about whether to ordain me.

One day he came to New Haven (he was a trustee of Yale University) and invited me to lunch. I reviewed my ideas about going to the School of Management. He thought that going to business school was an excellent idea and that I could have a major effect over time. I beamed.

"But you know, Bob," he said, "you are also very young. So I have a suggestion that you might want to consider."

I looked at him with hesitation.

"You might want to defer going on to study management until you have had some practice in ministry. If you move forward with your ordination, you could join a parish and learn about how to be a minister directly. And then, after a year or two, you could go back."

I thought about it. The school would accept deferments of up to two years.

"You would learn a lot about humanity in this role. When you are asked by people to participate in their weddings, their children's baptisms, their slow decline, and their funerals, you come to love people even more," he said, looking at me across the lunch table. "Listening and responding to people's questions week in and week out will deepen your knowledge and your wisdom." He paused. "But you should do what you feel called to do. It's just something to consider."

I went home and I did consider it, and I decided that he was right.

*

The end of my time at Yale Divinity School was marked by several momentous personal milestones. In March 1982 I became engaged to Dana Robert, a brilliant Ph.D. student in the Yale Religious Studies Department, who had grown up in Louisiana. In June I stood at the front of the local village parish of St. Barnabas in Irvington, New York, surrounded by friends and family, as Paul Moore laid his hands on me and ordained me a deacon. Following the order of service, I stood directly in front of the bishop, who looked straight into my eyes. He adopted his most formal voice and gave me my charge. My responsibility, he said, was "to serve all people, particularly the poor, the weak, the sick, and the lonely."

As I heard these words, I hoped that somehow, in some way, I might be able to fulfill this commitment.

In August, after more than nine months of searching, I moved to New York City to begin as an assistant minister— the most junior among five—at a magnificent and thriving congregation, Grace Church in Manhattan. In November, at a ceremony in Baton Rouge, Dana and I were married. In less than twelve months I had been transformed from an unmarried and unemployed student who could have ended up anywhere in the world into a married clergyman in one of the most amazing communities in New York City.

Nestled on the line between Greenwich Village and the East Village, Grace Church was a radiant force in the middle of the city. Designed by James Renwick in 1846 and built largely of white marble, the sanctuary was decorated with extraordinary stained glass windows, including one designed by Tiffany. The spire soared skyward on the corner of Tenth Street and Broadway. A few blocks west of the church lay Washington Square Park, originally the paupers' burial ground. To the east was the bustling East Village, filled with marvelous eateries offering everything from Italian pastries and Polish sausages to Hungarian stuffed cabbage and vegan stews. The streets were filled with students, immigrants, artists, service employees, and drug addicts. After we were married, Dana and I settled into a church-owned apartment on the top floor of Grace Church School, where I also served as the chaplain. My salary was tiny and barely covered our minimal needs, but we also had a free apartment with hardwood floors in New York City, prompting some of my visiting friends from college to ask if it was still possible for them to apply to divinity school.

Paul Moore had been right: the shift from being someone who thought about ministry in the abstract to someone who was serving a real congregation was transformative. Week after week I stood in the vast sanctuary with the great Te Deum window behind me, the long nave aisle leading to the rose window of the narthex before me. I regularly was invited by the senior staff to lead the service. On the table in front of me lay the polished silver paten and chalice given by generations now long gone, the white fair linen, the open prayer book, and the simple sacramental elements of bread and wine.

I would watch the people approach the altar rail—the young and the old, the strong and the frail, the honored and the despised, the joyful and the tortured. All would kneel; all would stretch out their hands to receive something that a material world could not give: hope, forgiveness, and deliverance. I was privileged to glimpse their eyes and see their longing assuaged, not through anything I had done but through some mysterious yet evident love that was reaching out to them.

There were many lovely aspects of serving in that community. The congregation was huge, filled with hundreds of young people in their twenties and thirties, many of whom had come to New York City to build their careers as actors, singers, writers, painters, and dancers. Their vibrant creativity pulsed through the congregation and made the services hum with energy. Among the older, more established members of the church I found a cross section of remarkable people, many of whom invited me into their homes. I met the widow of the great economist Adolph Berle, whose book on corporate governance had established the theory through which Franklin Roosevelt had created the Securities and Exchange Commission. I came to know many faculty and deans from the different colleges and universities. Other extraordinary and well-known people regularly visited the church on Sunday.

As I came to know the community and I was invited month after month to speak to the congregation from the pulpit, I found my voice. The school, which taught children from kindergarten through eighth grade, asked me to talk once a week to them about Bible stories. I quickly discovered that if I read the stories, the students immediately lost interest, but if I told them or we acted them out, they found them electrifying. And so I learned to narrate, without notes, the stories of Abraham and Sarah; Isaac and Rebekah; Jacob, Rachel, and Leah. I could talk about the life of Moses and the deliverance of the Hebrew people from bondage in Egypt. I could repeat the parables of the Good Samaritan, the Prodigal Son, and the Workers in the Vineyard. Eventually I brought this newfound skill into my sermons for adults, who reacted just as powerfully.

And, in a pattern that was now well established in my life, once I had settled in the community, I began to look more closely at the structure of the institution and to ask questions about its values. The early 1980s were the period when President Reagan and Congress were cutting funding for the housing and care of people with mental illness, and the trend was toward moving people away from large facilities and back into communities, which often meant out onto the streets. The United States economy was also in a recession. I watched with a growing feeling of outrage as the number of homeless people increased all around me. I noticed and worried about the wretched and filthy men and women who would sneak into the church garden for a place to sleep. When the rector of the church, a remote and difficult man, decided to evict them every night, I boiled with frustration.

One day the superintendent of the church posted a prominent sign on the grass that said "PRIVATE GARDEN." The notion that a church ostensibly committed to the poor was kicking people out of our manicured space infuriated me. I protested to my superiors and was overruled. So, in a rather juvenile act, I stole the sign late at night. A few days later the sign reappeared, this time bolted directly to the stone wall of the church. The next night I took a crowbar and started to pry it off again. In the middle of my act of vandalism, the number-two minister in the church, my friend and mentor Ken Swanson, heard the cracking noises and came rushing down with a baseball bat to scare away the crook. When he discovered me, he was both furious and amused. He scolded me but kept my secret.

As I entered my second year, the contradictions between the life of joy and ebullient generosity of the congregation and the misery of the people who rubbed up against our exterior walls bothered me more and more. Eventually my dismay focused on two questions: our refusal to tackle the problem of homelessness and the church leadership's unwillingness to examine the serious contradictions in our investment policies. I started to agitate about both.

To find out more about the problem of homelessness, I visited shelters and human service agencies around the city. One day I dressed in my most ragged clothes, put on an old down jacket, and pulled a wool cap tightly over my head, trying to approximate the standard outfit of a homeless man. The outfit did the trick; as I wandered the streets from morning until late at night, I was completely ignored by everyone. People refused to look at me. Fast-walking commuters steered a wide path around me. Vendors watched me with suspicion when I loitered in their shops. In the evening I lined up with hundreds of other men to have dinner at one of the city's biggest shelters. I could sense the dank and edgy depression that engulfed many of them. After dinner I waited on a dirty chair to be told by a social worker where I could spend the night. While I sat there, a fight erupted in the hallway. When I stepped out to see what was happening, two policemen were punching an unshaven man and throwing him up against a wall, shouting at him to stop doing something. When a small trickle of blood appeared from his nose, they backed off. I felt powerless and frightened. When I was finally called in and told that the only place for me that night meant taking a bus and then a ferry in the dark with hundreds of other men to sleep in a warehouse outside the prison on Riker's Island, I declined. I returned to my safe, quiet apartment and to my own bed, deeply shaken.

Every day I witnessed more human pain. I could not stop

thinking about a particular woman who sought refuge every day at the church. She used to sit, curled up in a ball, in an alcove just to the left of the front steps. The smell of urine and the clouds of flies were overpowering. Even when the temperature reached ninety degrees, she crouched down in a filthy overcoat. She never touched the small cups of water and juice I would take to her. At night or in a rainstorm she would disappear, but she always returned in the morning.

I tried to speak to her, but she never responded to anyone. Eventually I called social services and a New York City medical team arrived. Then her mouth opened. She cursed them violently and insisted she was fine and just wanted to be left alone. Later I saw her mumbling to herself and banging her fist lightly on the ground. For the next few days she sat there, and I continued to take her water, and one day she disappeared, never to be seen again.

During this period one of the readings in our cycle was the story of the rich man and Lazarus, from the Gospel of Luke:

> *There was a rich man who was dressed in purple and fine linen and lived in luxury every day. At his gate was laid a beggar named Lazarus, covered with sores and longing to eat what fell from the rich man's table. Even the dogs came and licked his sores . . .*
>
> *The time came when the beggar died and the angels carried him to Abraham's side. The rich man also died and was buried.*

The rich man, who is never given a name, discovers that he has been sent to a place of suffering where he can see Lazarus far in the distance, sitting at ease next to the patriarch Abraham. The rich man calls out, asking for help.

> *But Abraham replied, "Remember that in your lifetime*
> *you received your good things, while Lazarus received bad*
> *things, but now he is comforted here and you are in agony.*
> *And besides all this, between us and you a great chasm has*
> *been set in place, so that those who want to go from here to*
> *you cannot, nor can anyone cross over from there to us."*

As the words rang out, I kept thinking about the people huddled outside our church. Everyone in the building was concerned about them. But none of us knew what to do.

The church grounds contained several buildings, including a brownstone on Eleventh Street, and it occurred to me one day that perhaps the congregation would be willing to establish a small homeless shelter somewhere on the property. I raised this idea tentatively with the rector of the church and he showed no interest. I talked to Ken Swanson, and he responded with a mixture of openness and caution. I dropped the idea into conversations with the members of the vestry— the board of directors of the church—and they were largely indifferent. I quickly realized that to create a shelter I would have to back up a few steps. Members of the congregation would need to think about the problem, and then decide that they needed to find a solution, and then identify the solution

as a shelter at the church, and finally implement it successfully.

To begin this process, I approached the younger members
of the congregation and asked for their opinions. When they
expressed the same frustration and sadness, we talked about
what to do. Eventually several members of the congregation
decided that this was important, and they began to meet and
formulate a proposal. Ken decided to champion the idea with
the rector and the vestry, who continued to express reservations. The biggest objection came from the parents of the
schoolchildren, who worried that having homeless men in a
building near the school might represent a threat to the children
as they came and left. There were many other questions: Who
would welcome the homeless men every evening? Who would
remain with them overnight? What legal or medical responsibilities might we have? What training would volunteers need?
All of these problems had to be voiced and addressed. I kept
an informal list of important decision-makers and kept tabs on
their evolving views. Slowly, through the leadership of a growing number of people, the mood of the church tipped from resistance to acceptance. During my second year there, we finally
opened the shelter for twelve men, whom we always referred
to as "guests." People throughout the congregation signed up
as volunteers for different nights of the week. The nights that
I spent there were long and sometimes less than pleasant—
light came through the storefront window, the men snored and
grumbled in their sleep, their odors could be disturbing, and the
actual work of setting up beds, pillows, and blankets night after
night proved taxing. But as I lay there listening to them breath-

ing, I thought, For this one night they are here, and they are warm, and they have found shelter. For a few moments at least, Lazarus had been brought inside the safety of the gate.

*

In early 1984 I was nearing the end of my two-year tenure at Grace Church. On a beautiful spring day I traveled uptown for my annual visit to New York Hospital to review my blood tests and general health. For nearly three years people around the country had been dying of a terrible new illness, Acquired Immune Deficiency Syndrome, or AIDS, and doctors had recently developed the first test to see whether people had been exposed to the virus, known as HIV, that caused it. My concern about this had been tempered by the reality that I had already been exposed to many illnesses, including hepatitis A and B, through blood transfusions and I still seemed to be in strong health.

I entered the same building on the East River where I had been born and made my way to the sunlit offices of Dr. Margaret Hilgartner, the director of the hemophilia and medical oncology program. She was a tall, stately woman who had been my physician since I was five. Even though she was sometimes gruff, I liked her because she always answered my questions seriously. Once, while riding in a car with her, I inquired about her life. "Why did you become a doctor?" I asked. "In order to help people like you," she said quietly, and then looked out the window.

I was now sitting in her office. She carefully reviewed my test results and clinic notes.

"Your liver functions are slightly elevated, but that has been true for a long time," she said. "In general your joints are doing well." Then she paused. "Bob, as I think you know, we now have the capacity to test for the HIV antibody," she said quietly, "and we have your results. Would you like to know what they are?"

"Yes," I said.

She turned around and picked one great ledger book from a shelf behind her and dropped it on her desk. She then reached for a second massive book and put it beside the first. I had the feeling that I was looking across at the Book of Life and the Book of Death.

She opened the first book and ran her finger down a list of names until she found my coded number. She then opened the second, looking to match my number with my test results. She peered at it carefully. Then she looked up at me.

"The results show that you are positive," she said.

"What does that mean?" I asked.

"We don't know yet. It is worrisome. We will be watching your T-cell count and other blood numbers very closely to see if they drop."

"And if they do?" I asked.

"If they drop below a certain level, your immune system will be severely compromised and you will be considered to have AIDS. That would be very serious. We have no treatment right now. Until then, we will just watch and wait."

And then Margaret wished me well and I walked out. Later such a diagnosis was considered so frightening that it was delivered only in a highly controlled setting, with offers of support and counseling. But it was still early in the epidemic, and I was by myself, on a busy sidewalk in Manhattan, tentatively probing my feelings.

Thinking back on the thousands of transfusions and injections that had never led to any clinical impact, I decided that I would accept her advice. We would watch it carefully. I remember exactly where I was standing on First Avenue when I made a decision. I would not start acting as though I were terminally ill until the numbers started to show that I was terminally ill. Until then, I would live my life as fully as I had up until that point. I returned to our apartment and spoke to Dana. She did not seem to react, though I realized much later that the news set off a depth charge far below the surface.

In the months ahead, America plunged into a panic about the disease. I stood in a supermarket and spotted a magazine thirty feet away whose headline, in huge red letters, read "AIDS: NOW NO ONE IS SAFE." Frightened people demanded that the government quarantine everyone with HIV on an island off the coast of the United States. Violence flared against gay men. A family with hemophilia had their house in Florida burned down. The conservative writer William F. Buckley, Jr., proposed, half seriously, that everyone with HIV should be tattooed, prompting a furious public rebuttal from my father, a friend of his, who threatened to tattoo Buckley himself.

I watched as the debate swept across the country; as thousands of gay men struggled with the exhausting care and tragic deaths of those they loved; as families touched by hemophilia lost their beautiful sons, brothers, wives, and husbands; and as medical professionals showed what is best about our nation by committing everything they had to treating those with HIV.

During this period and in the years afterward I also asked myself a thousand times what would have happened if we had succeeded in holding hearings in the U.S. Senate about the viral contamination of blood products five years before anyone had heard of HIV. The hearings inevitably would have focused on the vulnerability of the system to widespread contamination with hepatitis and other viruses. Senator Jackson would have asked whether known viral inactivation techniques such as heat treatment could reduce the problem. Instead, because nothing happened, the products continued to be made and shipped without any antiviral treatment, so that when HIV appeared, it shot through the blood supply, and eight thousand mostly young men with hemophilia in the United States died.

I watched and I wondered, and late at night I worried. My time spent in the sanctuary of the church helped me gain perspective. I slowly began to accept that life, no matter how long we live, is achingly short. Every moment and every emotion is marked by fragility and meaning and grace. As we struggle together against all the currents that are carrying us relentlessly downstream, in the end our only real compass is love.

*

In my very last months at Grace the finances of the church captured my attention. As a junior member of the clergy I was allowed to sit in on the monthly meetings of the vestry. They gathered in the ornately carved office of the rector, a miniature Gothic library with soaring rib-vault ceilings and a magnificent row of mahogany bookcases. Every meeting included a report from the treasurer, which mapped out the monies spent and the monies received. To my surprise I learned that the church had a vast endowment—more than $9 million—which created a continuous cash flow vital to the physical upkeep of the historic building. I marveled that the church kept its basic financial information private from the rest of the congregation, from whom most of the revenues came.

As I thought about the endowment, I began wondering where the money was actually invested, and I approached the members of the finance committee. Their normally friendly smiles disappeared and they looked troubled. It really wasn't a question they could talk about, they said. The clear implication was that this was not a question for the clergy to consider, especially the *junior* clergy.

Yet I persisted. Eventually I obtained a list of the investments from one of the committee members, and as I studied it I was shocked. I don't remember everything that was on it, but it was clear that no one had ever asked whether the investments of the church aligned in any way with its mission. Red flags fluttered on every page. The church had large amounts of money in military contractors, including manufacturers of nuclear and other weapons. They owned shares of price-fixing pharmaceuticals, casinos, tobacco products, and alcohol. They held stock in companies that had substantial investments in

South Africa and other dictatorial countries. As I analyzed the information and the committee more carefully, it became clear what had happened. Most people on the vestry, including the rector, had no interest or expertise in investment, so they selected a few talented members of the group—bankers, trust officers, attorneys—to create a finance committee. The finance committee then placed the endowment with a conventional firm without restrictions. The justification was, of course, a version of fiduciary responsibility: the church, as a nonprofit, needed whatever revenues it could generate for its upkeep and its programs. The purpose of the fund was to maximize the amount of money it would receive. And if, to do so, the church ended up becoming part owners of and thus participants in enterprises that went against its own principles, that was not relevant. As long as the company's actions were legal, they were morally and financially acceptable.

From my previous work, I knew that this was problematic. I again began a small organizing campaign to bring this to the attention of the decision-makers of the church. I asked if I could go to the finance committee meetings; they declined. I suggested that they interview investment companies that excluded particularly disturbing industries from their portfolios and still made excellent returns; they demurred. I tried to put the topic on the vestry agenda; the rector refused. I brought it up over lunches and dinners with my closer friends; they politely but firmly changed the topic. After six months, I realized that I was being fully and effectively stonewalled.

I had only one option left: I could preach. This was a serious decision. On the one hand, as an ordained minister I had the authority to raise whatever issues I felt were important as long as I linked them to the gospel. The rector and the other clergy did not preapprove my words. The congregation was always attentive and respectful. At the same time, I knew that no matter how gently I phrased it, my words would infuriate some, including my boss. I still had a few more months in my contract, and I did not want to be tossed out. I also did not want to get to the end of my tenure and feel that I had never brought up the subject publicly.

I worked for weeks on my sermon, and as luck, or the spirit, would have it, my opportunity came when the passage assigned to my week was the parable of the rich young ruler.

As Jesus started on his way, a man ran up to him and fell on his knees before him.

"Good teacher," he asked, "what must I do to inherit eternal life?"

"Why do you call me good?" Jesus answered. "No one is good except God alone. You know the commandments: 'You shall not murder, you shall not commit adultery, you shall not steal, you shall not give false testimony, you shall not defraud, honor your father and mother.'"

"Teacher," he declared, "all these I have kept since I was a boy."

Jesus looked at him and loved him. "One thing you lack," he said. "Go, sell everything you have and give to the poor, and you will have treasure in heaven. Then come, follow me."

At this the man's face fell. He went away sad, because he had great wealth.

On a Sunday morning in early spring, I climbed the steps to the magnificent high wooden pulpit that rose next to one of the great stone columns of the church. The congregation sat down. I put my papers down and then looked out at the upturned faces of the hundreds of people in front of me, people of all ages, from many different backgrounds, almost all of them my friends.

I started with some lighthearted comments to put people at ease and spoke for some time about the passage, asking people to imagine this earnest young man, who came up to Jesus to ask him the most basic question of all: "What should I do?" Jesus, as he often did, quoted the Ten Commandments, the heart of Hebrew scripture. Yet the man was not satisfied—surely there must be something more! Jesus was touched by the man's intensity, his longing, and his passion. Perhaps he recognized some of the intensity of feeling that animated his followers or perhaps even himself as a younger man. Perhaps this person could become a new disciple, even a great one, fully dedicated to a life of compassion. If you want to deepen your commitment, Jesus told him, you must cut away the ties that are narrowing your vision, that are holding you back—in this case, your wealth. Rid yourself of that, and you will be completely free—free enough to join me on the greatest adventure in history. But this was not the news that the young man wanted to hear; which is why his "face fell." And it was not a move he was willing to make, so he walked away in sorrow.

The passage was intended not as a condemnation of all possessions but as a caution about their enormous power. This, I pointed out, was the only recorded moment in all of the New Testament where someone is directly asked by Jesus to follow him—and turns him down. If the young man had made a different decision, he might have been known for thousands of years by his name and celebrated for his love. Instead, his attachment to his wealth overwhelmed him.

The congregation looked appreciative. So far this had been a perfectly acceptable sermon, in both its analysis and presentation. I knew that if I stopped there, I would get the usual round of compliments at coffee hour, and that people would promise, with complete sincerity, to think about what I had said. I also knew that the effect of my words would fade almost instantly, and no matter how warmly my friends and colleagues embraced the ideas, it was unlikely that there would be any actions. So I kept going.

What was interesting about this passage, I continued, was that I had had a similar experience just recently at Grace Church. I had met a person who had approached me and asked, regularly and clearly, how to become more compassionate, how to deepen her commitment, and how to extend her faith into the world. Through these questions, I had come to appreciate and care for this person, and I had asked more deeply about her dilemma. She had inherited a substantial fortune, she said, but she felt constrained by it. The money was managed by a group of people who had every good intention for her, but they were preoccupied with making sure she became as wealthy as possible, so that she could lead a happy and safe life and give more and more to charity. She wanted to take another step into a life of Christian commitment, but she felt blocked by the cost of her beautiful home and her monthly expenses. She told her friends that she was committed to acts of generosity and peace, but when her bank statements and trust reports came every month, she felt discontent at her own failure. What should she do?, she had asked.

"This is an urgent question," I said, "because the woman in question is actually with us today, here at Grace Church."

Everyone fell silent and stared at me. No one stirred.

"In fact, she may be sitting next to you right now."

I could see them trying to remember what the person beside them looked like without actually turning their heads.

"What should we say to her? What would we advise?" I said quietly into the microphone. "This is important for us as members of Grace Church."

I waited. For a long time.

Then I spoke again.

"Because this woman *is* Grace Church."

The congregation seemed stunned.

In a few sentences, I laid out the dilemma of the gap between how we earned our money and how we spent it, how we invested our dollars and how we invested our time. I asked the congregation to raise the question, and I asked the leaders to answer it. For in that place, we were standing in front of Jesus just as much as the rich young ruler had been two thousand years before. I offered a prayer that we would make the right decision.

There I stopped. I picked up my pages and climbed down from the pulpit, steadying myself on the railings because I was shaking. As I moved back to my seat, I glanced at the rector, whose face was a wall of fury. When I sat down, a member of the choir turned to me and said, half in admiration and half in fear, "Well, *that* took guts."

At coffee hour the congregation registered their mixed emotions. Some embraced me with tears in their eyes. Others went quite far out of their way to avoid talking to me. When I went back to my apartment, Dana said that maybe I shouldn't have taken up such a controversial topic when I had only a few months left in my time at the church. I reflected on the reactions and decided, That's it. I will be fired within the next three days.

I was not fired, but I learned later that I had come close. The rector and some of the leaders of the church were deeply unhappy, and complained about my insubordination and arrogance. At the same time, a large portion of the church agreed that this was a problem that needed to be addressed, and they let the leadership know. Eventually the rector decided to let the clock run out on my contract. We rarely spoke after that.

And, sadly, the aftermath was similar to what happened at Ivy Club. Many people said they agreed with me and would work to do something about it. A few members of the vestry said that my rash actions had crushed the little seedlings of reform that had just broken through the surface. The rector maintained his stony silence.

Later that spring, after months of searching and application, Dana and I learned where we were headed next. She was within a few months of completing her doctorate, and she was hired to teach at Boston University's School of Theology. Instead of returning to the Yale School of Management, I had applied, as an experiment, to the doctoral program at Harvard Business School. I figured that if I was going to do all the coursework in business and economics, I might as well write a dissertation and be able to teach. To my utter astonishment, I was admitted with a full scholarship and told that I would also have to complete the first year of the MBA, the business school equivalent of boot camp.

In 1984, in the sweltering heat of mid-August Manhattan, Dana and I packed up our rust bucket of a car, bounced over the potholes, and crossed the city line, heading north to Massachusetts. In the months ahead, the question of the Grace Church endowment sputtered fitfully from time to time. The church eventually decided that it needed to protect the building more than it needed to worry about the portfolio. Over the next ten years, the parish lost much of its vibrancy, dipped regularly into the endowment of its principal, and gradually saw that sum shrink to insignificance. I am not sure what the perfect answer would have been for that community, but in the end the contradiction—and their inability to act—seemed unhappily to lead to a fading of both their fortune and their faith.

CHAPTER SIX

Up AND *Down*

The campus of Harvard Business School was built to inspire awe. The first time I walked around the campus in the fall of 1984, I looked at its massive and elegant buildings, its manicured lawns and pampered flora, and I thought of the Book of Exodus, as Moses stood before the burning bush and heard a voice that said, "Come no nearer; take off your sandals; the place where you are standing is holy ground."

On the fourth day of classes my marketing professor, Mark Albion, invited the members of Section F to introduce ourselves to one another. After all, he said, we were going to be spending an entire school year together in the same seats in the same room and we might like to know who our section mates were. As we went around the eighty-plus students, I counted two lawyers, eight consultants, nine accountants, seventeen engineers, and twenty-three bankers. Twenty-five of my classmates had gone to Ivy League schools, and thirty-five had majored in economics or business administration. Of those who had worked for large corporations before business school, four had worked for oil companies, three had worked for Procter & Gamble, three had worked for IBM, and two were currently on leave from General Motors. One fellow had been a captain in the Coldstream Guards and had led a platoon in Northern Ireland; another, a Marine Corps lieutenant, had served in Beirut at the time of the 1983 airport bombing. Also among our ranks were an architect, a Canadian ski instructor, and an Australian veterinarian. I was the only minister.

I barely remember what happened during those first weeks of school. Suddenly I'd been propelled from the Gothic halls of Grace Church and dropped into the world of business school, with its perplexing courses in marketing, accounting, managerial economics, and organizational behavior. Instead of relying on the language of theology, I was abruptly required to speak with an entirely new vocabulary, which consisted of phrases like *depreciation tax shield, cumulative probability, distribution curve, product cannibalization, net present value,* and *subordinated convertible debenture.* I also found myself designing a consumer and trade promotion campaign for Vaseline petroleum jelly.

The business school relies exclusively on the case method to teach its skills in the first year. This means that you are confronted with a detailed account (including reams of numbers and charts) of some business problem an executive is facing. You must begin by figuring out what's going on (often the most difficult task), then somehow derive a solution, and finally prepare a few remarks so that you will have something to say if you're the hapless student chosen at random to make the opening presentation the next morning. This analytical process is repeated with little variation approximately four hundred times during the school year, giving rise to a famous school adage: "First they scare you to death, then they work you to death, then they bore you to death."

*

After I had been at Harvard Business School for about six months, I realized that as much as I enjoyed everything I was learning, I needed a counterweight. While I was discovering new things about competition, I wanted to remember old themes from my life about cooperation. While I was becoming fascinated by the power of action, I wanted to recall the strength of contemplation. And while I was soaring upward into new realms, passing through all the grand hallways of Harvard and everything they represented, I wanted to stay rooted in a life attached to the ground.

I started looking for a spiritual home, where I could not just listen but also participate. In most regions, bishops maintain a list of "supply clergy" who are available to serve as stand-ins whenever a local minister is on vacation or needs to be away for personal reasons. I put myself on this list and soon found myself accepting invitations to visit different parishes around Massachusetts, from pocket Gothic churches in the suburbs to decaying wooden structures in the industrial cities and towns.

One day I received an invitation to go the following Sunday to Christ Church, a small church in Somerville, just across the river from Boston. The senior warden told me clearly that this was a one-shot arrangement, because the vestry was about to hire someone permanent. Fine, I said. She gave me the directions. When I arrived I was surprised to see that the sanctuary was only a few hundred feet from the elevated interstate highway. I was met by an ebullient, elegantly dressed woman in her sixties named Kay Emerson. Kay bubbled with hospitality; she showed me where to hang my robe, she introduced me to the organist, and she told me at least five times how pleased everyone was that I was there. How many people did she expect that morning? I asked.

"About ten," she said with a big smile.

"Ten?" I asked. That was unusually small, even for a tiny parish.

"Well, almost everyone else is on the vestry, and they are all at another church listening to the man we hope to hire as our permanent rector."

"Ah, well," I replied, "I understand."

When the service was over, I had a cup of coffee and greeted the few people who were there. Kay continued to express genuine delight.

"This is the most lovely place," she said.

Though the building was unassuming and the neighborhood run-down, I agreed with her. I can still remember standing at the entrance of the church, looking up and down the street at the long row of three-story apartment buildings known in New England as "triple-deckers." I took in the dirt ballparks across the field and the cars roaring by on the highway. For a fraction of a second I imagined myself returning to this place, getting to know the neighborhood, becoming part of the community, reminding myself of what was important in life.

"Well, thanks again, Pastor," said Kay. "We all loved your sermon! Goodbye!" She waved with winning sincerity, and I drove home.

That night I called the senior warden again. I enjoyed the visit, I said, and though I knew they didn't have any need for me, I was wondering if they knew of any other congregations that might benefit from a part-time person. No, she said, politely but firmly, she was not aware of any place like that.

"Let me know if you hear of anything," I said.

*

The business school gave tremendous weight (often 50 percent of one's grade) to classroom participation, and I realized early on that I would have to overcome my paralyzed silence. This was difficult, because my classmates were hurling new words and concepts around the room with ferocious speed.

Even more difficult than mastering the language was the challenge that I was an anomaly wherever I went. At business school, I was peculiar because I was a minister; with church friends and other ministers, I was equally peculiar because I was in business school. This tension between the life of faith and the life of business was exactly what I had gone to the business school to learn about, but I found it tricky to know how to act in class.

Once in a while I spoke up about what I thought were broader political or ethical issues raised by the cases. Was it really necessary to close this plant and throw hundreds of people out of work? Did any sane human being really want overpriced deodorant socks to be conveniently available in supermarkets? What effect might our extensive shampoo-marketing efforts have on the families we had targeted? Wasn't it possible that a highly profitable hospital chain might be earning money by excluding the poor? The class seemed to tolerate my outbursts but rarely supported them.

*

Four months after I visited Christ Church, I received another phone call from the senior warden. She sounded embarrassed but said that the other minister "hadn't worked out." "Would you be willing to come back for a few Sundays?" she asked.

"Sure," I replied. "How many do you need?"

She paused. "Sixteen," she finally said.

I gulped. That was a major commitment. I checked my calendar.

"I can do thirteen of the next sixteen," I said.

"Great," she said. "See you Sunday."

After the three months, the bishop appointed me to a longer tenure, thus launching my three years of service at Christ Episcopal Church and the adoption of my new home of Somerville, Massachusetts, where I have now lived and worked for almost three decades. Built at the turn of the twentieth century by farmers and fishermen who immigrated from Newfoundland, the church was solidly Protestant in its theology and practices. The members, many descended from those founders, worked as carpenters, insurance salesmen, boilermakers, steelworkers, teachers, house painters, and at every other trade at which one could make a living in a working-class city like Somerville. Some of the parishioners had come from very big families— ten children, thirteen children, *seventeen* children—and those children had grown up and married into other parish families. Many of them were thus related, mostly through the sisters and wives and mothers and aunts, who all had different last names but bore a family resemblance if you saw them sitting next to each other in the pews. It took me a long time to sort those connections out.

At the time I started at Christ Church, the community had shrunk. The entire budget for the year, including the small salaries that the organist and I received, plus the heat, hot water, electricity, insurance, Sunday school supplies, and the biggest category, repairs, came to a total of $39,000. If one looked at it through financial eyes, as I was being trained to do, it was hardly a going concern.

Still, we were rich in remarkable people. The church had a formal legal structure, with wardens, vestry, and others charged with making decisions, but as in many places the informal leaders had much more sway. One of the movers and shakers was the charming Kay Emerson and her quiet husband, Al, who walked faithfully behind her at every church event in his brown tie and tan jacket, watching her admiringly. Another formidable lady was May. May was in her late seventies and had come over from Ireland as a young woman; you could still hear her accent when she spoke, which was not often. She had raised a flock of children and was still cleaning houses from time to time when I met her. I had been there for several months when I stopped by the church one day and found May down on her hands and knees, polishing the hardwood floor and the gleaming pews. "What are you doing here, May?" I asked. "The same thing I do every Saturday," she said, pulling another rag out of her bucket.

She had endearing habits. During the warmer months of the year she often came to church in a floppy hat and sunglasses, and I could see that under her formal dress she was wearing a beach outfit. On such days she carried a large tote bag with slippers, sunscreen, a thermos, and several towels. Her plan was to attend church and then walk to the bus and take the subway to Revere Beach, a two-mile expanse of sand half an hour away.

There were other remarkable participants. Jim, a veteran who served as an usher, always brought his case of harmonicas so that he could accompany the hymns. A boilermaker named Roger, having heard that I didn't have any space to lay my papers or meet with parishioners in private, suddenly showed up one day with lumber, tools, and a few union friends. Within six hours they had framed out a section of the basement with wall and door and then carted in a desk and chair for my new office. I tried to thank them, but they all shook my hand, blushed, and faded away.

We began to attract a wide assortment of new parishioners. Since we were situated right on the largest athletic fields in Somerville, people sometimes walked in off the street. The residents and caregivers from a local community home for men with Down syndrome started to come every Sunday and within a short time indicated that they wanted to participate in the procession. From then on we had three or four mentally disabled people, wearing white robes and bearing great smiles, helping to carry the cross and the baskets of offerings at every service.

Over time, as people realized that the leadership of the church had settled down, they started coming more regularly and bringing their family members, friends, and loved ones. Soon my schedule filled with a roster of weddings and baptisms. It was not easy handling the demand for these personal connections and services while taking exams and writing papers as part of my responsibilities at Harvard, but I enjoyed it.

I also realized quickly that my parishioners were not moved by platitudes. The members of my congregation struggled with all the hard things that happen to a community under severe economic stress. They were out of work and unable to find new jobs. They had unusually difficult relationships with their families in all directions. They had limited education and opportunities. They often could not afford medical or dental care. Some turned to alcohol and drugs, or had spouses or children who did. Some of the women were struggling to free themselves from domestic abuse. Many marriages held on with the barest of threads or broke up completely. Most parents were trying to figure out how to raise children in a tough neighborhood. For the boys, the choices were to finish high school (if possible), find a trade such as carpentry or auto repair, join the military, and steer clear of the drug dealers. For the girls, the tasks were similar but even more stark: try to finish high school, don't get pregnant, look for a steady paying job (such as dental hygienist), and don't get married too young.

Occasionally my parishioners ended up in trouble with the law. Sometimes they didn't respond to a summons or have the right paperwork, or spent a night sobering up in jail, or got behind in their car payments or mortgages. Sometimes a member of one of the families would disappear and I would hear that he had been "sent up" for six months for driving while intoxicated or without a license. Single mothers struggled daily to protect, clothe, and feed their children. Young men got jumped in bar fights and then left town for a few months to let things cool down or to look for seasonal construction work in Florida.

As a small community, we did what we could, organizing food and clothing drives, referring people to leads on work, steering the most desperate toward social services or food stamps. The process of obtaining government assistance of any kind was itself interminable and disheartening, requiring a person to make six trips on the bus to the government offices (often in different locations) to pick up documents, fill out documents, get documents stamped, provide supporting documents, and get the final document of approval.

Despite the hard nature of many families' lives, they were often eager to build something beautiful at Christ Church. We had potluck suppers and holiday gatherings with lasagna and potato salad and Jell-O. Some of the children in my community looked too thin and tired, but they enjoyed running around the basement. A cluster of relatives chatted in the corners after services and tried to provide counsel, encouragement, and practical support.

*

At the business school I once tried to break out of the mold of class ethicist, just to see what it was like. We were discussing the problems of a men's cologne that was declining in popularity. I raised my hand and said, "It's all image and air anyway, so let's capture that air with a campaign built on the most expensive sort of snob appeal." The professor looked startled. "This from a man of your background?" The class laughed. I still don't know whether he meant it as a compliment or a reproof. In any case, I never again recommended something I didn't believe in.

As time went on I got to know the students better, and the more friends I made, the more I suffered from a dilemma. I found many of my section mates to be truly charming and thoughtful people. Despite the competitive pressures, mathematically gifted students willingly helped those who were struggling with numbers. When a student's mother and a professor's father died during the school year, the outpouring of emotion and donations was immediate and genuine. Some people even found time to participate in volunteer activities, such as becoming a Big Brother or organizing a blood drive.

I benefited all through the year from many people's friendship and assistance. One classmate picked me up and drove me to school for several days after I had hurt my knee. The night before the accounting final, another spent an hour with me on the phone and cleared up some of my questions, thereby enabling me to squeak through. And I was delighted when a dozen classmates from almost as many denominations formed a little Bible study and fellowship group. We met every Tuesday for lunch and talked about our backgrounds, our beliefs, and our doubts.

Some of my classmates offered me the opportunity to minister to them in moments of personal distress. One woman described her painful separation from her husband and daughter; another man told me in moving detail about the death of his father. On a few occasions people burst into tears as we talked, pouring out fears about their futures and frustrations with the relentless pressure of school. Over time many proved to be warm human beings, genuinely concerned about my well-being, and true friends.

Yet however thoughtful and kind the students were in private, in public they could sometimes be surprisingly unwilling to raise ethical objections to any business practice. During one case series, we studied a cold remedy that introduced no new medical features into the marketplace and whose advertising budget would represent 60 percent of its retail price. I decided to keep quiet and see what people would say. After the second day, nine people came up to me separately to inquire why I had not yet objected to this "piece of crap." I encouraged them to speak up, but they looked embarrassed. Even one professor remarked, again privately, that the product was terrible. But in three days of class discussion, no one openly objected.

And thus the dilemma: privately and personally the students were caring people, but publicly they became aggressive, even callous. In the fall we saw a movie on the coal miners' strike in Harlan County, Kentucky, and the sight of the overweight miners' wives brought wave after wave of cackling derision. When, in a discussion of textile workers in England, it was revealed that a woman who had sewn for twelve years for $2.50 an hour might lose her job, most of the class felt that she deserved to be laid off, since she was being paid too much.

Moreover, all day long the students talked about money. Discussions about money in such courses as managerial economics, control (the business school's term for accounting), or finance always had a clinical quality, as though money were a force with its own properties and principles, like electricity, rather than an instrument we use to express what we value. People forgot that the whole idea of exchange on the basis of price depended on a prior definition of possession; one could not sell what one had no right to own. And, as it became clearer to me over the years that followed, one often placed no value on things that had no price.

*

The most demanding and moving part of my job as a part-time pastor was visiting the seniors who could no longer come to the church. I had twelve such "shut-ins," as they were known, and I tried to visit them all every four to six weeks. This was a challenge, because I was living in Brighton at the time and it was a forty-minute commute before I could reach any of their homes. Yet I set aside the time to do it, and it was a profound and moving experience. I would study the map, drive to a person's residence, and carry in a little packet with a Bible, perhaps a small gift or a bit of food, and the necessary equipment for home communion. I would climb the back steps to the kitchen entrance, which was usually open. Once inside, I would call out the name of the person I was visiting and advance carefully through the house, not wanting to startle or wake anyone. Usually the person was in the same place, often a comfy chair in the kitchen, dining room, or living room. If the television was on, I would ask if I could turn it off, unless the person was completely enthralled with a soap opera. And then we would simply talk.

At the beginning all I noticed were the superficial aspects of each home: the memorabilia on the walls and mantelpieces, the decaying furniture, the uneaten containers of food, which I would often clean up and move into the kitchen trash. Some homes also had a strong and unpleasant smell, since many residents could not control their bladders or make it to the bathroom in time. I remember one cheerful woman who sat all day in her kitchen in a huge comfy chair that was soaked with her urine. She could reach everything from her spot— her radio, her refrigerator, and her cigarettes. She was always delighted to see me and received both news and communion eagerly. After such visits I often called the city's social services to request a professional evaluation of her needs. I thought she could not remain in that situation for long. People occasionally came by and cleaned her up, but then she sank into the chair again.

One couple in their eighties had not left their home for twenty-five years, and they had assembled a network, now dwindling, of people to pick up their groceries and other items. One day when I was visiting them, I saw an elderly woman vigorously vacuuming the dining room. When she finished, she took a mop to the floor in the kitchen.

"Who is that?" I asked Mr. Green, the husband.

"That's my aunt Maude," said Mr. Green, who was in his mid-eighties. "She comes to clean house every week."

"And how old is she?" I continued.

"Ninety-five," he said, without the slightest surprise. She had been cleaning up for him for decades, and he didn't find it unusual that she was still doing it.

My oldest parishioners told me amazing stories about growing up at the turn of the twentieth century. One of my favorites was Ruth, and though she had an occasionally sour view of the world and was as skittish as a cat, I could sometimes make her a cup of tea and get her talking about Somerville when she was a girl, around 1904. When she got going, she painted the picture of a bustling city, full of young men and women making their way in the world, shopkeepers and delivery boys chatting in their stores, politicians shaking hands, girls chasing hoops, and children sledding down snowy side streets. Her parents would send her at the age of five to the corner store, where she bought a quart of milk for seven cents and a loaf of bread for five.

Once while returning from such an errand she came across an ice man flogging his horse. Ice men dragged huge blocks of ice on sleighs and deposited them door to door through a special hatch built into the side of each house (our home still has one, now sealed off). In the absence of electric refrigeration, this arrangement kept food cool for days. The horse pulling this particular load was failing from the weight, the cold, and age or illness. The vendor, not wanting to lose his shipment, flogged it harder. Eventually, right in front of Ruth's eyes, the horse simply lowered itself to its side and died. Recounting the story more than eighty years later, Ruth relived it through a flurry of tears. "He was dead!" she cried in the tone of a horrified girl. "But still that man kept whipping him and whipping him! And there was nothing I or anyone could do!" She wept for five minutes. I sat there murmuring "I understand," watching the soul of a wounded child come flowing through the fragile and failing body of a very old woman perched like a bird across from me on a chair.

*

I also tended to the sick and the dying. I would learn through a phone call that someone had taken ill, and even though I lived forty minutes away I would head over to the hospital. Sometimes I made a mistake. Once Mrs. Green called just as I had come in the door: Was there any chance I could come soon to visit her husband? I would be happy to, I said, perhaps the following morning. Certainly, she said, though her voice lacked conviction. When I arrived at her home the next day, I discovered that Mr. Green had died; in fact, he had been dying when she was talking to me, and all she had wanted was for me to be with him at that moment. I felt I had let both of them down badly.

Death came month after month. Some were long anticipated and could be understood as the end of a long and rich life. I performed one funeral for a man from Newfoundland who had taken a job as a teenager on a North Atlantic fishing boat. On his first voyage, his captain received the call to go pull the frozen bodies of those who had died on the *Titanic* out of the ocean. There were also sudden tragedies that threw families into despair: car crashes, heart attacks, industrial accidents. One woman, who was tremendously overweight, had a fatal heart attack as she was preparing to go out with her family to celebrate her twenty-eighth birthday. At her service in a funeral home, the volume of tears from her friends and family made it almost impossible to finish. I tried to visit people whenever they were in the hospital. I knew as well as anyone how disorienting and frightening a hospital could be.

As my congregation aged, my visits changed. I was spending more time visiting people who were slowly dying of all the complications of old age. I memorized the location of all the pay phones on the street corners of Somerville so that I could call ahead to check with patients or their nurses. I came to know the parking lots, coffee shops, and wards of every hospital and nursing home. My job was simple but important: to offer words of comfort and encouragement to people who knew that they had started down the long exit ramp of the world. Some were resigned, some were terrified, and many were surprised, because their lives had moved so quickly. They wanted to tell me their stories, talk about why they wished they had talked to their parents or sister or husband one more time before some great separation, and told me about their fears of the medications and doctors that were slowly filling their lives like an incoming tide. I listened, and sometimes I brought them up-to-date on the news of the parish or gave them communion. I always prayed with them, which I quickly realized was not about my skill at finding the right words but about reminding them that there is nothing wrong or frightening about laying our desires, hopes, and fears before God.

I had six or eight people, mostly women, who shrank into drier and drier husks. They stopped moving and eating, they turned away from nurses who offered medication, they slept through most of our encounters. Sometimes they would wake and grab my fingers with striking power, as though they wanted to hold on to a few more minutes of life through my hand.

And then, one by one, they died. Sometimes, through some miracle, I was actually there, standing at their bedside while their breathing melted away and the room suddenly became filled with a dense, immovable peace. More often I would get a call that someone was failing, often at night, and I would do my best to put on my clothes and head out. When Kay Emerson's husband, Al, collapsed, I arrived just a few moments after his death. She was quiet but devastated. The doctors and nurses, having tried to save him, were wrapping up and stowing their equipment.

Al lay flat on his back, in the pajamas he had been wearing when the ambulance went streaking over to get him. Kay kissed his amiable face and shiny bald pate, and she tenderly stroked his cheek. When I held his hand, he was still warm, which does not last long after death.

*

To keep my sense of perspective, I tried, with uneven success, to maintain a regular discipline of daily prayer and Bible readings. And I tried to talk about what I was learning, though this proved difficult. Even the most well-intentioned business school student had trouble understanding my commitment to the parish, and most of the parishioners found it bizarre that I was spending any time at all in a business school. Over time it became apparent that underlying many of the discussions and decisions at the business school lay a philosophy of life that was shared but rarely discussed. The first article of faith in HBS doctrine was an unquestioning conviction of the economic and moral superiority of corporate capitalism. The basic justice and integrity of current economic arrangements were never publicly challenged.

More deeply, there was a belief that the free market always resolved any apparent disputes in a manner that benefited the most people. This powerful utilitarian idea is usually traced to the early economists Adam Smith and Jeremy Bentham, who preferred to identify themselves as moral philosophers. Smith's passing remark in *The Wealth of Nations* that the actions of individuals in the marketplace seeking to maximize their own advantage lead to benefits for everyone is one of the most misused texts in modern life. As Smith wrote, "[The businessman] intends only his own gain, and he is in this, as in many other cases, led by an invisible hand to promote an end which was no part of his intention. Nor is it always the worse for the society that it was not part of it. By pursuing his own interest he frequently promotes that of the society more effectually than when he really intends to promote it."

To begin, Smith meant this process to be understood within an entire system of compassion, which he referred to as "empathy," which is the topic of his earlier, similarly massive, yet never quoted book, *The Theory of Moral Sentiments*. Of equal interest is the changing nature of the concept of the "invisible hand" itself, which, as the economist Albert O. Hirschman points out in his book *The Rhetoric of Reaction*, began as a theological idea.

Human beings noticed all through history that events sometimes unfolded positively and sometimes negatively. One minute people were prospering, and the next they were carried off into exile by an invader. What was the deciding factor? they wondered. For many it was the hand of God, the powerful yet ultimately unknowable creator who organized human history according to an inscrutable logic. Later, in the eighteenth century, it became fashionable to talk less about a personal creator guiding history and more about the nature of "Providence." This was one of the preferred forms that George Washington and other founders used in referring to what they perceived to be the hidden power behind the unfolding American Revolution and the establishment of the United States. Within another generation, the "invisible hand" came into widespread use. As a social concept it remains powerful, because it relieves society—and particularly its leaders—from responsibility when things are apparently going poorly. Does it look as though an economy is damaging prosperity, people, and the planet? Then we should not trust that evidence! The truth, argue the proponents, is that no matter how poorly things may seem to be going, the overall trend must, by definition, be positive, through the power of the conveniently invisible hand. For those who are prospering, the evidence is self-evident, and for those who are suffering—well, they need to keep the faith that it will all work out for them in the end. The strange result is that while the doctrine of the invisible hand seems to encourage individual action—surely a good thing—it also seems to free our collective structures from blame if things do not achieve our collectively desired ends.

When taken up by a small but virulent group within the business community—and among some of the students—the consequences of this old and misapplied idea became an acetylene torch for a particular version of conservatism, one that later morphed into some of the core beliefs of the Tea Party movement. Government is always inefficient and something to be reduced, controlled, and mocked. Monopolies are bad if you are on the buying end but good if you can achieve them in your own industries (this is called building market share). American workers are fat, slow, and inefficient, and labor unions are a destructive force. Poverty and unemployment are the result of inefficiency and are primarily the fault of the poor and the unemployed. Almost any marketing or promotional campaign can be justified on the grounds that if a consumer actually buys the product, it must fulfill some sort of "need." Individual greed always aggregates to a larger good; therefore the rabid pursuit of materialism is without question a good thing. And if Americans didn't read the fine print on their purchases and got themselves in trouble on their homes, their credit cards, their loans, well, it was their own damn fault.

Eventually I got up the nerve to visit different professors to inquire about the curriculum and about their feelings on ethics in business. Many of them were eager to talk about the profound moral and philosophical problems of modern business. I even detected a certain frustration with some of the students' narrow focus. The more I talked to the professors and listened to their comments in class, the more it seemed that they had a definite mission they were seeking to fulfill through the design of the curriculum. Not only did they intend to turn out well-rounded general managers, but many of them also hoped by doing so to arrest or reverse America's decline as a manufacturing nation and world competitor. At the time—more than twenty years ago—the great anxiety was that Japanese firms had outperformed American firms because they had designed marketing programs that were more responsive to consumers, organizations that were more sensitive to employees, and factories that took seriously the contributions to quality and production offered by workers. The message to us was direct and simple: American managers must become more attentive listeners, more humble, more interested in the long term than the short term, and more devoted to the success of their companies than to their own careers. At the same time, in the same school, other faculty members were devising the systems of stock options and securitized debt that would soon pump the economy into a series of bubbles: first junk bonds, then technology, and finally subprime mortgages.

Although cooperation and long-term management were what the *curriculum* stressed, the *culture* at the business school emphasized the reverse. Students were graded on a forced bell curve, which rewarded people with prior training and work experience and automatically failed the bottom 10 to 15 percent in each class. The stereotype most admired by student culture was that of the "tough hands-on manager," someone who justifies his or her high pay by being the crisis solver, the problem fixer, the head basher.

In those days no one was more admired than the CEO of General Electric, Jack Welch. A graduate of the University of Massachusetts, Welch had risen through the ranks of GE as a tough, take-no-prisoners manager who demanded that the businesses under his supervision become first or second in their markets or they would be sold. When he became the CEO of GE, he fired so many people that he became known as "Neutron Jack," a reference to the atomic weapon that killed humans but left the buildings standing.

On one occasion Welch came to the Harvard Business School campus to address the eight hundred first-year students in Burden Hall. He gave a rousing speech about leadership and toughness, and he was rewarded with a huge wave of applause. All the faculty who had a relationship with GE, or who hoped to be permitted to write business school cases about its decisions, sat in the front row and beamed. Then came time for questions. Several people asked him versions of the same question: How did it feel to be the greatest business leader in the United States—or possibly ever? Welch took the questions with blustery self-confidence, sharing his platitudes about the need to be a fierce competitor.

Then I raised my hand and he called on me.

"Mr. Welch," I said, "last week a coalition of major religious organizations known as the Interfaith Center on Corporate Responsibility held a press conference identifying the twelve companies that have played the most significant roles in supporting the South African government through loans and strategic goods and services. General Electric was near the top of that list. What are General Electric's plans for the future of its relationship with the government of South Africa?"

I knew Welch wouldn't like it, but I had designed the question to be as fair as possible. What surprised me was the reaction of the other students. As soon as I said the words "South Africa," a large number of students in the hall began to hiss at me. Their hissing intensified as I completed the question. They were clearly outraged at this breach in courtesy; how dare I ask such a question of the greatest executive in America after he had done us the honor of visiting the school?

Welch shifted his weight forward like a fighter and actually stepped closer to the bottom of the section where I was standing. He then launched into a long, largely incoherent explanation: of course GE opposed South African racism and its leaders weren't really supporting it that much; in fact, they had put some practices into place that would ultimately help their black workers; and besides, the company couldn't get into judging how its products were actually used. His statement was full of factual inaccuracies, and I was gearing up for a follow-up question that would force a little more honesty out of him. But when he finished, I could sense the hostility surrounding me. So I let his flimsy answer stand, and I sat down.

*

Over my years at Christ Church and Harvard Business School, Dana and I settled into an evenly paced life in a small apartment on the edge of Boston. She completed her dissertation, became an assistant professor at the Boston University School of Theology, and taught some of the most popular courses at the school. As she rose in her field and I came nearer to finishing my degree, we faced a major decision: whether to have children. We had held back for more than four years because of uncertainty about my precise HIV status. During that time we scoured the country for more information, and we designed a detailed process of counseling, heart-to-heart conversations, and spiritual reflection to decide whether this was something we would pursue. Doctors really couldn't advise us, except to suggest that in their best judgment, as long as I seemed so healthy, the risk was likely to be small. I was strong and my immune system was completely intact. We decided, after a process of reflection and prayer, to go ahead. We had two sons, Sam and John, in quick succession, in 1987 and 1989, and everyone tested fine. Dana and the boys were completely healthy. We rejoiced and decided to stop there. Though my own long-term fate remained uncertain, I settled into a period of deep contentment that I had been blessed with such interesting work and such a beautiful family.

*

At no time is the emphasis on individual success and achievement more evident than in the frenzied winter mating season when recruiters arrive at the business school. During that period I occasionally went to the business school in a suit because I had appointments in town immediately after class, and each time my section mates playfully inquired if I had "given in" and decided to interview with McKinsey or Goldman Sachs. "Come on, Bob," one good friend of mine said. "Those consulting jobs look pretty good, don't they? Wouldn't it be fun to tell other companies what to do? Wouldn't you like to make thousands of dollars a week for a summer job?"

But whenever I started to fantasize or worry about "all the money I really deserved to be making," I would look through the Bible, and the fever would leave me. The morning before my finance exam, the lectionary pointed me to a passage from the First Letter to Timothy which combined words of warning with words of support:

> *We brought nothing into the world; for that matter we cannot take anything with us when we leave, but if we have food and covering we may rest content. Those who want to be rich fall into temptations and snares and many foolish harmful desires which plunge men into ruin and perdition.*

The love of money is the root of all evil things, and there are some who in reaching for it have wandered from the faith and spiked themselves on many thorny griefs.

But you must shun all this, and pursue justice, piety, fidelity, love, fortitude, and gentleness.

The spectacle of hundreds of students desperately searching for work was not without irony when one remembered the ease with which these same students proposed to shut plants and fire workers who had been employed for twenty-five years. The students, however, did not consider themselves to be in the same league as workers; they had become managers. Having put up tens of thousands for tuition and earned a degree from Harvard, they felt they deserved a job.

Over my years at the business school I gradually came to understand more about the creative power of American business and I became less critical about some things. I understood, for example, how extraordinarily difficult it is to run a business, how many complex and divergent parts—finance, marketing, sales, production, distribution—all have to be coordinated. And I came to believe that there is much that is good about a few people coming together, pooling their resources, and trying to provide a service or a product for which they earn a return on their investment. In other words, I have become a huge fan of small business.

For the serious person of faith who commutes between a church on Sunday and a corporate job on weekdays, who is drawn by the hope and joy and freedom of the gospel yet must live amid the rules of the marketplace, the only choice is to cultivate an active, brave, and responsible capacity for moral choice, often in defiance of social and institutional pressures. Church leaders fortunate enough to have money to set aside cannot escape the difficult question of how to invest those funds in a manner consistent with their beliefs. And on a global level, no person who professes that all human beings are beloved children of the same God can be complacent in a world where billions live in subhuman poverty.

As the years progressed, I came to realize that the most profound question posed by a place like Harvard Business School is one common to every human endeavor: What greater goal or God are we individually and collectively called to serve in life? I found myself wondering constantly what the school was really teaching. Some might argue that it communicates a useful and value-free body of knowledge, in the same way that a school for auto mechanics communicates certain functional skills. But an alternative view occurred to me when I returned to a gathering of the members of Grace Church and someone welcomed me back as "one of our three seminarians who have gone off to study." Another speaker commented, "I know we live in Orwellian times and war is peace, but I never thought I would hear Harvard Business School described as a seminary. But I don't know. Maybe it's true."

*

Though the hours were long and demanding, I did my best for my congregation, for my family, and for the doctoral program

I was in. My mind and intellect were learning volumes of valuable information from Harvard University, while my heart and soul were growing at Christ Church. For one thing, I realized that no matter how hard we worked to provide for one another as a congregation, there were certain physical problems that a small community could not solve by itself. We could provide support and comfort and companionship, but not medical care and housing and a decent job. We could help people through their personal crises, but we could not educate their children, clean their streets, protect them from crime, or offer them a park in which to play. The voluntary commitment and extra effort made possible by a loving community was an important piece for some of our members, but the line between health and disease, education and deprivation, homes and homelessness, unemployment and a job, was not drawn by us. It was drawn by the government, as part of a basic promise to the American people that each person would receive the elementary requirements to build his or her own version of the American Dream. Government might seem like an abstraction to people who can provide everything from their own abundance, but to people in a city like Somerville, access to the building blocks of a decent middle-class life meant the difference between poverty and prosperity, misery and joy.

Second, I learned that no matter how good people's intentions might be, we are all stretched and easily overwhelmed. Being the part-time pastor of a church that had no resources required me to make hundreds of phone calls to terribly busy, pressed people who had virtually no money and asking them to take on some responsibility for the church—serving on the vestry, reading the lessons, teaching Sunday school, visiting the sick, leading the stewardship campaign. At first I thought they would jump at the opportunity, but I didn't fully appreciate how complicated and stressful most people's lives were in trying to make ends meet. I learned to ask the question and wait for a polite and somewhat embarrassed no. What was amazing to me in retrospect is how many people said yes.

Most churches have leadership retreats during which a small group of involved individuals, including the clergy, go away for a day or two to discuss the direction and priorities of the church. Christ Church had never done such a thing, at least within living memory. I called a friend of mine at a church about ten miles away, and he offered to provide meeting space and to prepare lunch for us.

"How many people will you be?" he asked.

I did some quick tabulations in my head.

"I would say between twelve and fourteen," I answered.

We agreed on the date and I publicized the event. I phoned every person and I was delighted that my numbers seemed about right—I had twelve people who were planning to come.

I made a list of passages we could discuss and of challenges facing the church. I wanted to urge us to move past our worship together and into offering more services for the people in the community. I wanted to develop more leadership skills among my small but talented group of committed participants. I was excited about everything that was about to happen.

We were to meet on Saturday morning at the church and

then drive together to our host. The night before, I got two phone calls at home. One person had been called away to work. Another couple gave me some sketchy reason that they couldn't attend, which I didn't push too hard to explore. Well, I was down to nine people plus me—still a good showing.

When I arrived the next morning, there were two notes on the door from people in the neighborhood who said that for various reasons they could not come. Now I was down to six. I unlocked the door and saw the light beeping on the church answering machine, indicating two messages. My heart sank. Sure enough, two more people had discovered urgent reasons—at this point I no longer cared what they were— why they couldn't come. They were, of course, very sorry. Very, very sorry. Would love to do it next time. Hope that you have a great time and look forward to hearing about it.

At this point I blew my stack. Four people. Twelve had said they would come, and now I was down to four. How could I plan for the future of the church with four people? I stomped out into our tiny little garden and marched in a circle around our single scrawny rosebush.

At that point Tony Cucinotta, a hardworking plumber who undoubtedly would have preferred to rest after a long week, showed up. I couldn't hide my anger and disappointment with the others.

"They told me that they would do it!" I shouted. "They said that they would come and then they backed out. They committed to being here for each other and to help build the community for all of us, and they dropped the ball. I am upset for myself, because I worked hard to put this together. I am embarrassed in relation to the church that has prepared twelve lunches for us. But more than anything, I can't believe that all these people couldn't stick with their own commitments."

Tony watched me carefully and stroked his chin.

"You're upset because they are not doing something they promised," he said.

"Yes!" I replied.

"Well, Bob," he said with a wry smile, "now you know how God must feel."

And with his words, my anger evaporated and we laughed long and hard.

CHAPTER SEVEN

Force AND *Freedom*

We may wish to abolish conflict, but we cannot get rid of diversity. We must face life as it is and understand that diversity is its most essential feature. Fear of difference is dread of life itself.

—MARY PARKER FOLLETT

Every morning when we awake and look at the news, we see almost everything through a single powerful belief. The institutions and arrangements of the world are fixed, we think, and we must operate within their boundaries. All the normal structures of life in America—the limits set by our Constitution, the laws constructed by our legislatures, the rules and practices established by our most powerful institutions, including our corporations, and the social standards and practices reinforced by daily life—seem to be made of steel.

These structures of society represent a body of received wisdom that developed over many years and that we now silently accept. They function as the rules of the road for our collective behavior. Only rarely, within a few communities or at key historical moments, are our practices ever fully debated from first principles.

Yet clinging to old answers is not always the right solution for difficult problems. By doing so we face the danger that our institutions will slowly slide away from our aspirations, that they will grow in rigidity without reason. We can become so accustomed to everything around us that we find ourselves increasingly trapped by the past and by forms perpetuated without function. It is as though we started off swimming in a pool of water into which time pours a slow stream of powdered cement. Without being aware, we find ourselves swimming against a thicker and thicker liquid, which gradually slows us down, dries out, and imprisons us forever.

Though we may firmly believe that we are stuck, the truth is that European and American society has been changing constantly for centuries. Every generation has faced a new social and political reality with new problems, new rules, and often new freedoms. For many people, such questions seem abstract, far removed from the demands of daily life, but every now and then the opportunity arises for people to design from scratch a new organization, or perhaps an entirely new social system. In the United States, this happened over the fourteen-year period from 1775, when Americans began armed resistance to British authority, to 1789, with the ratification of the Bill of Rights. In those rare historical moments, people get to step back and ask: What is the best way to organize our lives? To achieve our goals?

One of the greatest experiences of my life was the opportunity to observe at close hand the complete transformation of a whole country—South Africa—as it remade itself from a nation driven by force and fear into one that now embraces the goals of liberty, justice, and equality. The transformation was not without difficulty, and the result has not been perfect. Yet seeing the complete reconfiguration of a nation unfold before my own eyes without widespread violence permanently changed my view of what is possible. I saw that the goals and structures of society can be controlled by the values and dreams of its citizens, and not the other way around.

*

In the late 1980s I finished my doctorate at Harvard Business School, which included a long technical dissertation that examined how some of America's largest investors—pension funds, church and university endowments, and foundations—made decisions about their investments in South Africa. While working on this project I read hundreds of articles on every aspect of this debate, and I pored through archives in different institutions and libraries around the country. Oddly, though everyone I interviewed told me that it was an extremely important topic, no one seemed to be working on a single comprehensive book on the subject.

One afternoon as I was nearing the end of my dissertation, I stopped by the office of Rosabeth Moss Kanter, one of the business school's most creative and distinguished faculty members. She asked me where I was in my studies, and

I told her that I was nearly finished. I then shared with her the mystery of the missing book. It was peculiar, she admitted, but maybe the comprehensive book could only be written by a person with the right background. I thought about my own training—as a historian and an economist, as a minister who understood the passion for justice, and as a business school graduate who understood the mechanics of foreign investment—and I found myself wondering if perhaps this wasn't the perfect opportunity for me. I mentioned this to her.

"Well," she commented, "I have always felt that life is too short for small projects."

And that's all it took. As I walked out of her office, I knew what I was going to be doing for the next few years: writing a full account of the struggle for racial justice in the United States and South Africa in the era of apartheid.

After a valuable stint at the Kennedy School of Government in a new and creative program on ethics, I was hired by Harvard Divinity School to teach a range of crossover courses (the kinds of courses I'd dreamed of at Yale Divinity School) on the divestment movement, on how to create social change, on how communities in conflict could be reconciled. The dean encouraged me to establish a new venture called the Project on Business, Values, and the Economy. I settled into a small office on the second floor of an old carriage house on a back street in Cambridge. I organized monthly lunch discussions for faculty from across the whole university to discuss everything from the decision to close a major auto plant in Michigan (taught by an associate dean at the business school) to the pope's encyclical on capitalism (taught by a leading professor at the divinity school). Soon I had a flood of passionate and brilliant students, mostly from the divinity school but also from across the university and the region.

I set out to assemble a project of research on South Africa. I began collecting information across many topics: foreign investment, American politics, civil rights, and African history. I developed files on U.S. presidential policy toward Africa from the time of Harry Truman through Ronald Reagan. Because many South Africans passed through Boston and Cambridge, I made a point of asking to meet them and interview them. One of the couples, André and Maretha du Toit, became dear friends. André was one of the most prominent political philosophers in South Africa, an Afrikaner who had left a post at the University of Stellenbosch because of his fierce opposition to apartheid and was now teaching at the University of Cape Town. His wife, Maretha, the daughter of an Afrikaner minister, had also rejected the entire system of racial injustice, and she radiated enthusiasm and affection toward everyone around her, including me. The two of them took me under their wing, and soon I was regularly eating dinner in their small sublet apartment with South Africa's most distinguished leaders, white and black, as they stopped in Cambridge for a few days.

After a few years Dana and I realized that we would both benefit from a research year in another country, and we picked South Africa. I had already been there several times for research, and it seemed an ideal time to go as a family. Nelson Mandela had been released from prison two years before, and the exiled members of the African National Congress had returned to South Africa to begin the arduous process of negotiating a new constitution and a transition of power. Dana and I each applied for a senior Fulbright scholarship, which would give us just enough money to move there for six months with our young boys. In 1992 we received the award, and we scheduled our departure for early January 1993, a few weeks before Bill Clinton was to be sworn in as the new president of the United States.

The day arrived in late December, we handed over our keys to our house sitters, and we boarded a series of flights that would take us to the southern tip of Africa. When we arrived in Johannesburg, we traveled to the home of a gentle Afrikaner couple, Jacques and Carol Kriel, whom I had met on an earlier visit. It had been in their kitchen that I first encountered South African gastronomic peculiarities like rooibos tea, made from the red leaves of a South African bush, and the strangely delicious yeast spread imported from England known as Marmite. They also fed me mielie pap, a cornmeal porridge, and rusks, which are slightly sweet hunks of dry raisin bread served and dunked at teatime. It was in their home that I first noticed that though South Africans never have screens on their windows, there are remarkably few bugs at night. It was in their garden that I first saw great African birds sweep through the sky and watched monkeys pick through a compost heap. Flanking their driveway stood two six-foot-tall jade plants, magnificent tropical plants that had taken decades to reach that height.

As we were driving along their street I noticed the tight security around most of the homes. Every residence was surrounded by a tall fence, and every gate announced that a security company known as "Armed Response" or some other frightening name was protecting the premises. Everyone had added two or three feet of stones or fencing or razor wire on top of their walls—a physical barometer of the fear rising among Johannesburg's white elite. The one exception to this neighborhood trend was the Kriel home, which had such a low wall that a child could have hopped over it in a flash.

I asked Jacques about his wall, and he said that he did not want to make it any higher, even though they had already experienced a theft. Several months before, a group of thieves had entered their home while the Kriels were asleep and stolen the only two pieces of electronic equipment they owned, their television and stereo. Their immense dog, Bassie, a mixture of Great Dane and Rhodesian ridgeback who stood as tall as a pony and normally emitted a giant bark that struck terror into newcomers, had slept through the whole incident.

I asked Jacques whether things were becoming better or worse. Crime was definitely worse, Jacques replied, but on the whole this was a better South Africa than I had seen on my earlier trips. "You turn on the television and you see the neo-Nazis and the Communists debating each other," he said. "That was inconceivable a few years ago. So we are seeing an improvement."

*

Though our eventual destination was Cape Town, a thousand miles to the southwest, where we had rented a home, we took a few days to drive around the area, including a visit to the nation's capital, Pretoria. The great irony of South Africa was that its discriminatory structure had arisen because of the ardent desire of a particular ethnic group for freedom. The Afrikaner people, who numbered barely more than a million, were descendants of the original Dutch settlers who had built their homes in the Cape Province. After a hundred and fifty years, as part of the wars with Napoleon, the British navy sailed into Table Bay and took control. The British quickly established their own language, laws, and customs as the rule of the land, and they treated the Afrikaners as second-class citizens with regard to land and political rights. Afrikaners had a long history of importing slaves and subjugating local African groups, and the British insisted that they could not punish or kill their workers without proper judicial review. Eventually the Afrikaners decided that they had had enough, and they organized the "Great Trek," an enormous wagon train in which thousands of people moved all their portable belongings across the huge desert to find a home outside British rule.

These "Fore-Travelers"—Voortrekkers—settled in Pretoria, nearly a thousand miles to the northeast of Cape Town, only to find, to their horror, that within a generation the discovery of gold in nearby Johannesburg prompted the British to come rushing into their new republic in search of new wealth. The Afrikaners wanted freedom; the British responded by conquering them with force. At the end of the nineteenth century, they sent an imperial army to crush the resistance of these farmers, or Boers, in a brutal war of attrition aimed partly at the civilian population.

This experience burned for decades in the living memories of the Afrikaners, who swore that one day they would regain control from the British and be free to do what they wanted with "their" land and "their" blacks. A huge wave of nationalist rallies began in the 1930s, and some of the major Afrikaner leaders, including one future prime minister, were jailed by the British for favoring the defeat of Britain by Hitler. After the war, however, the Afrikaners finally achieved what they wanted: they won a majority in the whites-only election for Parliament. Led by a charismatic and demented professor named Hendrik Verwoerd, they wiped out the remnants of British law and changed the voting structures to secure permanent power for themselves.

To make sure they had no future opposition of any kind, they constructed a comprehensive legal and police system to control the majority black population. Africans were denied the right to vote, to own businesses, to travel without permission and identity documents, to live anywhere except in designated areas, to speak in public or to protest, to attend universities, or to resist the government in any way. They were to remain in a permanent state of "apartness," or apartheid, excluded from every chance to participate and to prosper. And thus the Afrikaners' desire to preserve their culture in freedom and their generational grievances against the English justified the creation and enforcement of the most modern and aggressive system of racism in the world.

To see some of the monuments of this troubled history, we drove north on a major highway cutting through green and yellow rolling terrain dotted with industrial parks that reminded us of east Texas. We went first to the Voortrekker Monument. Built in 1938 as a neofascist shrine to Afrikaner victory, the monument is one of the most visually powerful and politically controversial structures in the country. We climbed a hundred steps to the central chamber, where Afrikaner settler mythology is laid out in a large frieze around a central crypt. The building is built so that each year on the sixteenth of December—the date in 1838 on which five hundred Afrikaners rebuffed an attack by thousands of Zulus—a shaft of sunlight streaks through the window and illuminates a stone table at the center. The table resembles a sarcophagus; carved deeply in the top are the words "*Ons Vir Jou Suid Afrika*": "We (Are) for You, South Africa."

The place evoked many sentiments. It bothered me that the settler imagery seemed so familiar. If the bearded white men had been wearing Pilgrim hats or cowboy boots, I wondered, would I have found it as appalling?

We climbed more steps to obtain a sweeping view of Pretoria. There my mind shifted back to college. During my senior year, in the same spring as my bout with the eating clubs, I had also become deeply involved with the student divestment movement to protest apartheid. We had spent weeks marching in front of Nassau Hall, the student administration building, shouting, "Princeton—Pretoria! Break the connection *now!*" During my final months at Princeton, hundreds of students had joined this daily protest. I had admired the top student leaders greatly and wondered how they had acquired so much detailed knowledge about the business connections of the university. We handed out flyers and took buses into New York City to see one of our classmates testify against apartheid at the United Nations. In April 1978 more than two hundred students, including me, had seized and occupied Nassau Hall and spent twenty-four hours singing songs, holding teach-ins, and sleeping in the corridors to provoke a response from the university trustees, which never came. That incident, as much as any, launched me on a lifetime of study and activism on corporate and investment policy.

As the sun beat down on my little family nearly fifteen years later, I thought how far away Princeton seemed—a small town now locked in the snows of an opposite season on the other side of the world. The claim that there had been a connection between Princeton and Pretoria had at first seemed unlikely. It had required squeezing a long and complicated set of relationships into a single binary pair. "It's not that simple," administrators and trustees had told us in the 1970s, and in one sense they had been right. And yet they had also been wrong. Firms from around the globe—from the United States, France, Great Britain, West Germany, and Japan—had provided South Africa's white leaders with large amounts of money and technology to build their racist state. When I was at Princeton, nearly four hundred American companies owned subsidiaries in South Africa. Even though these firms never accounted for more than a fifth of South Africa's direct foreign investment, they dominated such key sectors as electronics, automobile manufacturing, financial services, and petroleum refining and distribution. Dividends from these companies had flowed into Princeton's bank accounts, and some of their executives sat on the university's board of trustees. The connection had been real.

*

Over the next few days we moved to Cape Town and settled into the house that would be ours for nearly six months. Our new home came with a station wagon, two dogs, a gardener named Nelson, and a maid named Tembisa. It was surrounded by a high wall and included a swimming pool just off the kitchen entrance. By the standard of South African whites, this was not particularly affluent, and I realized within days how seductive the whole environment could be.

My goal in South Africa was ambitious. After years of archival research and interviews in the United States, I had come to South Africa to complete the other side of the equation. It was one thing to write about apartheid as an idea, but what was it like for the people, black and white, who lived it? I was trying to assemble, as diligently and fairly as possible, a thorough explanation of how and why South Africa had both started and ended its modern system of racial domination. With this goal in mind, I made an ordered spreadsheet of the 120 places I wanted to visit and people I wanted to see in the 180 days I would be in the country. I jumped on this list immediately, making arrangements through phone calls, letters, and visits. E-mail didn't exist in South Africa, and many people were too busy to make commitments over the phone, so

I found that the most effective way to get something done was simply to show up at an organization or a person's front door.

To maintain our daily life, we enrolled our boys in the local Catholic school, where they wore uniforms and ran around with mostly white children in a neocolonial setting. John, who was three and a half, exuberantly made friends and seemed oblivious to issues of race. I began hearing about his friendship with a little girl in the class, and one day, when I picked him up, I asked him to point her out to me. He pointed to the only African girl in the room.

"There she is," he said, smiling. "She's the one in the purple dress!"

Samuel, five and a half, was blond and serious. One of his favorite pastimes was explaining plate tectonics to perplexed adults. He became popular in his class because he could help other children learn to read. He was nicknamed "Home Alone" because his blond hair and American accent reminded the other children of the actor Macaulay Culkin, who had starred in that movie a couple of years before.

Soon we settled into the easy lives of a white South African family. Our house was comfortable and food was cheap. The boys swam in the pool and made friends, and we went to dinner parties. People invited us over to their cookouts, and the men drank beer around the grill and chatted while the owner waved away the smoke.

From this bubble of privilege, it was harder to learn what was happening in other parts of South Africa, even parts that were physically nearby. Our maid, Tembisa, came and went and mostly resisted my efforts to engage her in conversation about her life. One of the few questions she asked me was whether South African blacks who traveled to the United States were forced to live in black townships during their visits. I tried to explain that although there was segregation in America, in which people of color lived together in poor neighborhoods, it was also true that a visiting black man could stay in a hotel in the center of the city if he had the money. She didn't quite believe me. I eventually learned that her father had died in one of the government-created potato famines and that Tembisa was struggling to support three children.

Our gardener, Nelson, appeared once or twice a week but then stopped appearing completely. We got word that he had fallen ill with tuberculosis, but he was out of our reach in one of the remote and largely invisible townships that ringed the city. When I made an effort to try to find him, I was cautioned by our physicians against doing so, because tuberculosis in South Africa was highly contagious and often fatal.

To add to the illusion of comfort and to the surrealism, the weather constantly reminded us of California. The sky was almost always blue, and the sun sparkled on the bay. Dana set up a place to do her research on the main campus of the University of Cape Town, and I drove into the city to an old prison that had been renovated to become the University of Cape Town's Graduate School of Business. The route passed a small game reserve near the base of Table Mountain in the center of the city, so I often found myself on a smooth highway zipping past the South African antelopes known as kudu grazing in the blond grass while I listened to the Beach Boys.

In many ways, the Graduate School of Business of the

University of Cape Town also seemed familiar, having been modeled on modern business schools around the world. It had all the accoutrements of respectability: well-organized MBA and executive programs, semicircular classrooms with printed name cards, carefully drafted case studies as part of the curriculum. The place was spanking new, and it also exuded potential.

Yet as an outsider, I immediately sensed peculiar and disturbing undercurrents. I couldn't help wondering what kinds of grim things had happened in those cells now turned into whitewashed offices with jaunty modern furniture. I found it distasteful that the school joked about its legacy. On the walls one found framed lithographs of the construction of the building by prison labor, early maps of Cape Town with "Breakwater Jail" clearly marked, and even a "wanted poster" for a black man named John Brown. The poster was so popular that the school had put it on a T-shirt that was sold in the gift shop, a move that struck me as tasteless at best, racist at worst.

Even though the business school saw itself as one of the leading institutions in the "new South Africa," and even though most of my colleagues thought of themselves as far more liberal than almost anyone in the country, there was one glaring problem: there were virtually no black students. When I asked, I was told that in the MBA program of over one hundred there was *one* African. The curriculum at the time showed no evidence that the country was undergoing significant political change or that there was an immense population of black Africans and "Coloureds" (members of a distinctive mixed-race community who spoke Afrikaans rather than

English) who would soon be released into an economy in dire need of advanced management training.

Even though the country was in the midst of rapid change, I encountered highly racist attitudes almost everywhere I went. Traveling on a boat across Table Bay, a friendly teacher from a technical university asked me where I was from. When he learned that I was from the United States, he immediately launched into the standard white South African line about how good it was I had come to see the country, because the problems were so much more complex than the international media suggested. Within five minutes he had delivered an unusually compact version of a speech I heard many times. There would never be peace, he said, because South Africa is made up of too many different nations, cultures, and "people groups" (a tip-off to his conservative religious views); blacks were uneducated and couldn't think for themselves, so democracy was an impossibility; if there were elections, blacks would vote on the basis of who could intimidate them the most; and Coloureds were terrified of blacks. I tried to slow him down with a few polite rebuttals—"Perhaps, but don't you think that . . ."—but he was undeterred. He seemed so eager to have the approval of an outsider that he didn't seem to hear that I was not giving it.

For a few minutes he offered his own pet solution: that South Africa should be divided into three nearly autonomous areas which would cooperate only on foreign policy and defense. "What would be the racial composition of these three areas?" I asked. He looked at me blankly, as though it were the first time he had ever considered the idea. Then he launched into a bigoted description of the Zulus in Natal.

Many new friends insisted that the question, *of course*, wasn't about race; it was about maintaining excellence. When I asked whether there might be a significant component of bias in the determination of standards—and even more in the testing to see whether those standards had been achieved—people looked at me with confusion and distress. Indeed, as I traveled through the privileged parts of South African society, particularly in business and the universities, I met scores of well-intentioned, intelligent, generous people who seemed to have little understanding of their own country. They read the paper and traveled abroad and wanted Nelson Mandela to succeed. But walking through these circles, I often felt that I had entered a beautiful restaurant where everyone was laughing and clinking glasses without being aware that the whole establishment rested on the rim of a rumbling, smoking volcano.

*

I did not spend all of my time in white South Africa. I also went to places where black and Coloured people lived, in many cases only a few miles away and yet a world apart. Stretching out across a long sandy plain, Cape Town had two kinds of slums. The first was the township, a slightly older and more established community, with tiny cinderblock houses, a few stores and gas stations, and the occasional church. Garbage blew aimlessly through the streets while people did their best to collect the necessities of life and walk to the bus stations that would take them to their jobs in the white sections of town. Up in Johannesburg, the white authorities had set aside a portion to the south which they named the "South West Township," whose name was shortened into a kind of acronym: Soweto. By the time I visited South Africa, Soweto had grown to more than a million people. The comparable townships in Cape Town were Nyanga and Langa.

The second kind of slum was the squatter camp. In these areas hundreds of thousands of people, many seeking work and housing but denied both, set up makeshift shelters in whatever form they could find: cardboard, plastic garbage bags, old crates, strips of burlap, and sheets of corrugated tin. Families jammed themselves into spaces about ten feet square, side by side, stretching mile after mile after mile. In Cape Town, one of the squatter camps, known as Crossroads, contained a million people and sprawled across the Cape Flats around the airport. The terrain looked as though a huge bomb had exploded, throwing up dirt, rocks, and concrete in every direction, and then people had moved in and built hovels on top of the rubble. In the middle of these oceans of humanity, the police and military had set up intimidating forts of concrete and lacerating barbed wire and watchtowers armed by soldiers with high-powered assault rifles. Parked behind the walls were rows of Casspirs, greenish-yellow armored personnel carriers that carried soldiers out among the black community and served as the main tactical weapon of the government during the suppression of township violence. Most of the young boys killed during the uprising in 1985 and 1986 had been shot like rabbits by soldiers inside the protective steel womb of the Casspirs.

*

In many ways it was easy to be moved or outraged at what I saw in South Africa, but I was self-aware enough to realize that I was seeing things that also existed, with less intensity, all over the United States. I was making the effort to explore the contradictions of a foreign country without ever having made the same attempt in my own. There are many places in America that are just as invisible to most Americans as the squatter towns are to South Africans.

Still, while I was there, I wanted to see things with my own eyes, and that desire took me all over the country. I took a special tour of a South African gold mine which plunged me two and a half kilometers below the surface into a dark and sweltering world where I was invited to try my hand at the hydraulic drills, march through miles of subterranean tunnels, watch the building-sized machinery crush and filter the rocks into powder, and witness the final pouring of molten gold into ingots. Thousands of men labored around me in tunnels stretching for miles in every direction, and yet even when I was down in their midst, I could get only the tiniest glimpse of the harsh conditions that humanity imposed on them in search of the ultimate symbol of human greed. Later the Chamber of Mines treated all the foreign visitors to a fancy lunch, to which they invited some of the white mine supervisors. The supervisors were delighted to be out of the mine for an afternoon, and after they had each downed three or four beers, they happily shared their wisdom with me, particularly with regard to the differing characters of the thousands of African men still working miles below us as we ate.

"The Shangaans, the Zulus from Mozambique, they're the best," said one man, grabbing me by the shoulder to get my attention and waving a big finger in my face to make his point. "The Xhosas, they are big, strong, and stupid. The Zulus are hard workers, but you have to watch your back. The Tswanas and the Sothos, they're shit. They are all political, all ANC— they always want something, and they cause trouble." Then he laughed congenially and slapped me on the back, as though I, as a white person, certainly knew what he meant.

Given the rage and fear that gripped people of all races in every corner of the country, I wondered how anyone could rise above this cauldron of misery and hate in order to create a genuinely new nation. While Africans yearned desperately for rapid progress, whites worried about everything they might lose, and the members of other ethnic groups—the Coloureds and Indians and other peoples of South Africa—felt that they were inevitably going to be caught in the crossfire. Yet through all of this, leaders like Nelson Mandela, only recently released from prison, and even his counterpart, F. W. de Klerk, the head of the apartheid National Party, had decided to guide their nation into a new future, to move forward with a measured, careful, and inspired commitment to creating a democracy. They were joined in this effort by thousands of people trying to contribute to peaceful change. I traveled the country seeking out the exceptional men and women who seemed able both to sense the terrible longings and fears around them and to patiently chart a new course.

I came to know and love Barney Pityana, one of the martyr

Steve Biko's closest friends, who had been imprisoned, then eventually left for England, where he became both a lawyer and an Anglican priest before returning to South Africa. He eventually became the head of the Human Rights Commission and then vice chancellor of South Africa's largest university. I met and sometimes had dinner with Albie Sachs, a brilliant Jewish lawyer who had joined the ANC as a young man, had argued for the creation of a nonracial democracy, and was nearly killed by a car bomb in Mozambique. The blast blinded him in one eye and tore off his right hand. He later became the equivalent of a justice of the U.S. Supreme Court. I spent a long time in conversation with Desmond Tutu, the archbishop of Cape Town and winner of the Nobel Peace Prize, who had been vilified in the press as "that black Communist bug" and yet laughed with joy at the thought of the new nation being born. I met theologians, business leaders, teachers, community activists, and men and women who had been tortured or whose family members had died in prison or been shot on lonely roads at night by the security forces. I even met the president of the country, F. W. de Klerk, at a reception at the U.S. embassy. I told him that I was studying the effect of sanctions on the South African economy, and he asked me pleasantly if I was finding good data.

"It depends on the industry," I said diplomatically. "As you know, Mr. President, some industries are not currently permitted to release such data." (It was, in fact, still a crime for South Africans even to ask.)

"It will be interesting to see what you discover," he said.

This was my moment, and I seized it. Plucking up my

courage, I asked him point-blank, "Did your religious convictions play an important part in your decisions of the last few years?"

"Yes, yes!" he said emphatically, to my astonishment. "People keep calling me a pragmatist, but that's not right. If anything, I have to struggle with not being a fundamentalist. I belong to a church that takes the Bible very seriously. I am always looking, always searching, for the basic foundation, the underlying *principle*, from which one can build an idea of the future, from which one can construct an action plan. As a Christian, I have always been preoccupied with this question of principle, of what is the right thing to do."

For a moment I found myself speechless, staring at a man who was both the head of one of the most brutal regimes in the world and someone actively seeking to bend his country's history toward justice. How could I ever communicate such human contradictions in my writing? I wondered.

The most elusive person in the country was, of course, Nelson Mandela. After he was imprisoned, in 1962, his name and his face were officially banned from every South African publication. I had visited South Africa just before his release, and since there were no known pictures of him since he had been in his forties, the newspapers had hired artists to imagine what the seventy-two-year-old man would look like when he stepped out of prison. The South African government even decided to minimize the shock of his sudden launch into freedom by driving him around the area in an unmarked car, and on more than one occasion they pulled over and allowed him to go into a corner store to buy a newspaper.

Many remember the image of Mandela finally leaving prison on February 11, 1990: the tall, gray-haired man dressed in an impeccable suit, surrounded by triumphant assistants, walking with measured steps toward the gates of the prison, hand in hand with his long-suffering wife, Winnie. The image was carried live on television around the world. He had spent nineteen of his more than twenty-seven years in prison in a tiny cell on barren Robben Island, surrounded by rapid ocean currents and marooned just six miles offshore yet in full view of Cape Town's beautiful cityscape. After Mandela was released, I had the opportunity to visit his old cell in the company of the United States ambassador, Princeton Lyman. The building was still being operated as a prison at that time, and the authorities had to clear the prisoners from that cell and from that block when we went. When I walked in, my heart rose to my throat. It was a tiny room, no more than eight by ten feet in dimension, with a small metal bed and a tiny desk. The ambassador and I could not fit inside at the same time. I tried, in the few moments I was there, to project backward through nineteen winters and summers, to wonder how anyone could have survived in this space without going mad. I looked at the thick, heavy bars that covered the window and realized that all I could see was a naked stone courtyard.

Yet Mandela had somehow remained internally free. After he left the prison, he instantly became the central figure in the South Africa story and an international beacon of hope. During my visit I arranged to meet with his personal attaché, a woman named Barbara Masekela, who later became minister of culture and ambassador to France. She had traveled with Mandela when he began to make foreign trips to support the transition to democracy in South Africa. She told me in particular about a recent trip to Tanzania, when thousands of people were lined up along the roads to the cities to catch a glimpse of Mandela. "We were traveling in an open four-wheel-drive truck," she said, "and if you listened carefully, you could hear the people saying 'Mandela, Mandela.' As soon as they saw him they said his name, as though they couldn't believe it. So as we drove, we heard the name, *Mandela, Mandela,* wave after wave, repeated like an echo. Everyone who sees him for the first time suddenly realizes 'There he is,' and for that moment they are alone in history with Mandela."

"They are alone in history with Mandela." The phrase struck me as profound. Most of us think of history as something that other people, important people, make. We read about it, we follow behind it, we bend to its force. We are like small boats tethered to the stern of an ocean liner, bouncing around in the boiling wake as we are dragged along. But for those standing on the bridge, there is no history; there is no wake; there is only the sea stretching forward, only the destination ahead. Everything happens in the present; there is no need to look back. Masekela said that this was something that amazed her about Mandela, Sisulu, and the others who endured Robben Island. "One cannot help looking at him," she said, "and thinking that he was robbed of his life. Yet he never mentions this. It is the same with all of them—Sisulu, Mbeki, all of them—they never allude to the fact that twenty-eight years of their lives were taken away. They are just going forward with what has to be done now."

And as she finished her sentence, the door behind her popped open, and Mandela himself stepped in.

"*Madiba,*" she said, using the name of both affection and respect favored by his inner circle, "this is Dr. Massie from the United States."

Mandela stepped forward and shook my hand, beaming. The only thing I could remember to say was that the secretary to the dean of the Harvard Divinity School, an African-American woman named Gwen Hawke, had made me promise that if I ever met him, I would give him her personal expression of gratitude.

"Please thank her very much," he said. "Tell her I find her words most encouraging."

And then he turned, papers in hand, and went back to his office, signaling to Masekela to join him. I watched the door close and realized that the camera I had brought all the way from the United States just in case anything like this ever happened lay unused in my briefcase beside me on the floor. But whether or not I had the visual proof, I had for a moment been alone in history with Mandela.

*

When asked about the personal adulation that was his constant fare, Mandela was always scrupulously modest. "I serve as one small human peg on which the nations of the world hang their admiration for the African National Congress," he told one

American television reporter. In some ways it was true. Mandela had not made the revolution himself. Yet he also enabled some extraordinary things to happen because, not unlike another tall, reticent figure who played a key role in the birth of his nation—George Washington—Mandela gave subtle approval or discouragement to many impulses that had been let loose in the complex negotiations for the transfer of power.

For several years South Africa had been slowly and steadily working to define both a new form of government and a pathway that would enable it to get there. It was a devilishly complicated problem. The Afrikaners had felt brutally oppressed by the British, and the key to their decision to impose apartheid was not so much that they hated blacks—though many of them did—but that they wanted to design a structure under which their political, cultural, and economic dominance would never be threatened by anyone. As a result of this insecurity, people of other races in South Africa had been systematically excluded and brutalized. Property had been stolen, families annihilated, futures destroyed, parents and children killed. Though the violence was mostly on the part of the white government, Africans had sometimes fought back, stealing cars and shooting their drivers, tossing hand grenades into truck cabs, and sweeping down on farmers and settlers in the depths of night. The South African military and police routinely tortured and murdered civilians, planted bombs, and drove opponents of all races off the roads into fiery deaths in ravines. To shatter the political unity of their opposition, the South African government also set up stooge governments in fake

black "homelands," where petty tyrants, wallowing in government cash and using their guards and militias to demand
tribute, drove around in Mercedes and lived in luxury while
their enforcers dragged men and women from their homes to
beat and kill anyone who dared to object.

At about this time, my son John asked, "Are there any
dinosaurs in the world?"

"No, John," I replied. "There are no longer any dinosaurs
in the world."

"Are there any ghosts in the world?" he asked.

"No, there are no ghosts," I said.

"And Daddy," he said, his face filled with earnestness and
anxiety, "are there any *monsters* in the world?"

Suddenly I felt a pang of anguish. What I said was "No,
John, there are no monsters in the world." But the voice in my
mind said, "Only human ones, John. Only human ones."

Later that night John's voice came back to me—"Are there
any monsters in the world?"—as I tried to fall asleep. A rapid
stream of images from the last few months roared through
my mind: the elderly white farmer strangled by thieves and
left in a cupboard for days; the four township women lined up
against a wall and shot through the back of the head; the hol-
low eyes of abandoned urban children begging for coins; the
humiliated faces of the men who shuffled to our door pleading
for food and work; the man screaming as he burned to death in
the trunk of his car just a few miles from our home.

Suffering of any kind is terrible, but needless suffering is
worse, and deliberately inflicted suffering is a specially hid-

eous evil. The world abounds in deliberate, calculated cruelty wrought by rational persons on other persons. As the images rocketed past, my intellectual explanations and psychological defenses deflated and I felt only horror. John's voice and mine intermingled, ringing like bell changes from a distant cathedral: "Are there any monsters in the world?" "Only human ones"—again and again, until I fell asleep.

*

F. W. de Klerk and Nelson Mandela, and the thousands of people who pulled together to build a new nation, woke every morning during this period and looked out at millions of people still boiling with deep historical grievances, reacting to current incidents of violence and gripped with fear that the future would only be worse.

How did they make progress? They designed a disciplined process and set clear expectations. Though their organizations had been enemies and were still in competition with each other, they found ways to work together. They promised that all the issues would be discussed until people around the country felt they had been heard. Accordingly, hundreds of groups pulled together in forums and debates and lecture halls and meeting rooms to announce their preferences. In retrospect, I can hardly believe how much time was spent talking. There were "national forums" on housing, on education, on a bill of rights, on a free press, on the role of the judiciary, which would sometimes draw in two or three hundred people for several days every few months. Everyone got the chance to speak, and then to speak again, and to keep going, on and on, until people finally decided that the issue had been talked to extinction. This didn't mean that every effort led to agreement, but it certainly meant that most people felt they had been given the chance to speak their minds.

As in the United States during our own revolutionary period, every political decision carried an attached theory. The natural tendency in political systems toward tyranny meant that there had to be checks and balances. Clarity of national purpose and efficiency of execution meant that there had to be a strong central government. Yet regional and ethnic differences needed to be acknowledged through smaller political boundaries, which Americans call states and South Africans decided to name provinces. The South Africans allowed their eyes to roam over the other constitutions of the world, and they adopted features from those of the United States, Canada, and Sweden. They worried about how to balance executive and judicial power. They debated for years about how to identify and preserve the individual rights of citizens.

Every morning I would rise from the bedroom that looked out over a piece of Table Mountain, descend to the kitchen, make a cup of coffee, and open the newspaper to read documents that reminded me of the Federalist Papers. In how many places in the world could one follow daily debates over fundamental constitutional issues at the moment of a nation's birth on the front page, in the editorials, and even in the comics?

And in how many places in the world could one see an entire nation looking for a method that would enable the country to mix justice with mercy? In most cases in which a war has taken place, especially a civil war, the victors expend their newfound power in hunting down and punishing the leaders of the other side as well as the perpetrators of the worst atrocities. The battles may no longer be military, but the sense of outrage and blame continues apace, with one side seeking openly to force the other to acknowledge their mistakes and pay the price.

South Africa had endured so many terrible acts over so many years, many of them in secret, that the truth, even after decades of efforts, thousands of prison sentences, and tens of millions in expenses, might still never be known. The need for justice in the most egregious cases was never doubted, but eventually the South Africans realized that an even deeper political and, more important, *human* need might be met through the creation of a commission that sought not punishment but truth, not vindication but understanding.

Thus the South Africans, borrowing from earlier experience in Chile, created the Truth and Reconciliation Commission, or TRC. Cochaired by Archbishop Desmond Tutu and made up of leaders of all races and backgrounds, the TRC was given clear instructions. Anyone who had committed a crime could be freed from prosecution by stepping before the commission and offering a full and complete confession. If a person offered only part of the story, he or she could still be charged and punished by a prosecutor for the unnamed part. Only through a full explanation of what had happened would the hand of justice be stayed.

The process was only just being organized during 1993, and it was deeply controversial. It sounded to some like cheap forgiveness. Wiser heads pointed out that for a nation to begin anew, the secrecy needed to end. And the designers and participants understood a deeper truth: that in many cases, the families of victims wanted more than anything to know what had happened and why. Prosecution was only one tool to obtain that information. And now that South Africa was changing, many of the perpetrators were feeling troubled by their own decisions and actions. Over the months and years ahead, hundreds of men and women came forward to ask their questions, tell their stories, and bow, figuratively and literally, before the horror of what had happened. The testimony produced moments of excruciating human suffering and of remarkable courage. The process created the opportunity for those who had done something grotesquely wrong to ask their victims and their listeners, in all humility, for what they knew they did not deserve: forgiveness. It did not happen in every case, and perhaps it should not have happened in some, but when it did, it unleashed a healing power that took everyone by surprise and often left them in tears.

*

Though events continued to unfold at a blistering pace, with major decisions about the future of the country being made every day in the paper, our sojourn as a family drew to a close. I attended the memorial service for the assassinated South African Communist leader—and surprising peacemaker—

Chris Hani in Desmond Tutu's cathedral in downtown Cape Town. After the service I joined an initially peaceful march that turned ugly as the police surrounded the central square with soldiers who carried military weapons loaded with live ammunition. I walked past burning cars and smashed shop windows into a huge rally, where I found myself caught between dancing, chanting, angry young African men and the white soldiers fingering the triggers on their machine guns. I realized uncomfortably that, unlike in the movies, there would be no background music to warn me when the shooting was about to start, and that I could there and then be killed by a bullet without ever being aware of what had hit me. I gradually withdrew and found my way back to my car. Eventually the protest ended without a massacre.

A few days later the negotiating parties took a major step and committed themselves to a firm date—April 1994—for the first countrywide elections to determine the future government and president. That move gave all the citizens a specific focus for their concerns and activism. The energy in the country shifted to making rules for the elections and analyzing the politics of various races. In the midst of all of this, Dana and I and the boys packed up and returned to the United States, at the end of June 1993. The weather in Cape Town was becoming cold and rainy as the region entered its dark winter period. Within a few weeks, however, we were sitting on the porch of an airy summer cottage in the Catskill Mountains, where we sometimes went for part of the summer. There was almost no news about South Africa, even in the *New York Times*. It was as though we had awoken from a long, remote, and impossibly detailed dream.

＊

The most surprising outcome of my extended stay in South Africa is that soon after I returned, I began to think about running for office myself. Up until that point I thought I had lived by a decision to work for change, but not through elective office. My experiences with Washington, with the Vietnam War, with Watergate, and even with my own short clash with the pharmaceutical industry had convinced me that politics was a corrupt, venal business, and that to step forward into political life was to risk both disappointment and contamination.

South Africa had changed this view. Of course there were huge complexities and unpleasant realities in that country, and the participants ran the gamut from virtuous to foul, with every intermediate blend. Yet it had been moving and exhilarating to watch a whole nation tackle its most basic problems, define its bedrock principles, and then put those into place. By flying practically around the world, I had come to a new appreciation for the democracy that had been born on our own soil here in America. When I returned to Massachusetts, two questions immediately presented themselves: Was I ready for politics, and was politics ready for me?

I assembled a group of close friends for a weekend and told them that I wanted their advice and spiritual scrutiny. That I felt a pull into politics was not in doubt; what needed to be answered, in personal terms, was more subtle: was this a temptation or a calling? Was I pursuing this purely as an act of ego, or was there some deeper, more worthy motivation? My friends spent several days putting me through detailed questions, and I then spent months pondering the decision. Eventually I came away with a clear sense that I should try.

The decision to become a candidate did not automatically open a pathway within politics. In the fall of 1993 the state representative and state senate seats were solidly filled. The mayor of Somerville showed no signs of stepping down. To run for office, you need an office to run for. After examining the options carefully, I decided that there was only one: the office of lieutenant governor.

At first blush, this seemed to many like an absurdity. I was thirty-seven years old, I had no political network, no personal fortune, and no name recognition. I was not an athlete, a movie star, or an astronaut. Moreover, the lieutenant governor had an unclear role in politics and in government. I was often asked the same two contradictory questions by different reporters. First they would ask, "What makes you qualified for the second highest constitutional office in the state?" and second, often asked immediately on the heels of the first, "Why do you want this do-nothing job?"

My response was always the same: I wanted to reinvigorate democracy within both the Democratic Party and the state. I talked about all the things I had cared about for years—health care, social justice, jobs, poverty, and the excitement of directing our own future. To some, I undoubtedly seemed naive. Slowly my words began to seep out and affect people. People were tired of a political agenda that included nothing but anger and division, that talked only about crime, welfare, and taxes (the three big topics that year), and they wanted to hear something and someone new.

I visited the chair of the Democratic Party, state senator Joan Menard, and asked her how many people were planning to run for lieutenant governor. She knew of only one, she said, a state representative. Is it possible that he would be the only person and might simply end up with the nomination? It could happen, she said. Did she know of anyone else who was thinking of running? No, she replied.

Surprised by my interest, she spoke with fairness and respect. As I left her ornate office, I thought to myself, "There really is a hole at the center of the Democratic Party. And maybe someone like me could fill it."

I visited the Democratic issues convention in October with Bob Colt, a well-known political operative who worked for the attorney general. After seven hours of shaking hands and greeting skeptical people, I felt sorry when they began streaming out of the stadium.

"But I haven't met everyone!" I complained to Bob.

"Oh, you are hooked," Bob said with a laugh.

Starting with two graduate students, no money, and no campaigning experience, I began my run. Soon I had raised a few thousand dollars and we opened a tiny office on the Cambridge-Somerville line. The technology could hardly have been more primitive: we had one computer, which we used to keep track of donations. We were a few years away from the explosion of the Internet and the technological revolution that changed American life and politics so dramatically. It took us months before we could finally afford a single portable telephone that would travel in the car. We had no e-mail and no GPS. But we had volunteers, and we had spirit, and more than anything we were having a great time.

The weather in early 1994 was brutal; I ended up driving to events through sixteen different snowstorms. I visited restaurants, union halls, factories, VFW posts, as well as innumerable living rooms for house parties. I was delighted that I was able to persuade my old friends Peter, Paul, and Mary to come to Massachusetts to hold a concert for me. They arrived in late February to perform in a hall that held 1,200 people. The morning of the concert, twelve inches of snow dropped onto the streets and cut our attendance to about 700, so that even though the trio had offered their services for free, the overall expenses outweighed the revenue. But it produced a huge return in credibility and enthusiasm for the campaign.

In early March, as my campaign was reaching fever pitch, South Africa suddenly popped back into my life. I received a formal invitation to serve as an official international observer at the South African elections, which were going to be held at the end of April. I presented this opportunity to my campaign manager Lynda Wik and the other members of my campaign staff.

"What would this mean?" they asked.

"It would mean I would fly to South Africa for a week."

My field director, Barbara Opacki, objected strenuously. "The state convention is only six weeks after that!" she protested. "If you don't get fifteen percent of the vote at that gathering, you won't even be on the ballot. You need to use every breathing moment to be calling delegates to introduce yourself to them in the hope that you can round up at least five hundred votes!"

I said I was still inclined to go.

"You also need to talk to about fifty reporters to see if a few more of them will write about you before the convention," my advisers continued. "How are you going to get any coverage if you're in another country?"

I felt uncertain. On the one hand, they might well be right. I had set off in pursuit of this unlikely nomination, drawn other people in, organized a strong campaign, and challenged the party establishment. It didn't seem sensible to pack my bags and leave for a week in the middle of the fray.

At the same time, I had been following the transformation of South African apartheid for nearly twenty years. I had just been there during a key constitutional period. With this invitation I was being offered a front-row seat and a particular way to help.

I went home and thought about it carefully. The next morning I returned. The South African elections were a key moment in world history, I said, and I wanted to participate in them. My team shook their heads with bewilderment but accepted the idea. We prepared as best we could for what seemed like a long absence.

I flew from Boston to New York City and walked through the terminal toward the sixteen-hour flight to Johannesburg. As I was entering the boarding area, I heard an announcement over the intercom.

"Would Robert Massie please pick up any white phone to speak to information?"

Bewildered, I found a phone and picked it up. The operator informed me that my campaign was urgently trying to reach me. I phoned my campaign manager.

"We just got a call from one of the local television stations. They've learned that you are going to South Africa and they're wondering if they could do an on-air telephone interview with you tomorrow when you arrive. They don't have a reporter on the ground, and they would like to get someone to describe the situation."

"Sure," I said, startled.

"Here's the number," she said. "And don't forget!"

I arrived in Johannesburg the next day and made my way to the downtown skyscraper that lodged the offices of the International Electoral Commission, which gave credentials to observers. The security was tight, so the line of people waiting to be admitted snaked across a vast public plaza surrounded by parked cars. The morning's newspapers were filled with threats from neo-Nazi parties that they intended to disrupt the elections through any means necessary. All around me police were stopping and searching vehicles for bombs. Standing out in the open under a gray sky, staring at rows of unoccupied cars parked closely to the electoral nerve center of the country, I found myself praying for the line to hurry up. When I eventually made it inside, I breathed a sigh of relief.

I received my credentials, including a special blue cap, a photo ID badge to hang around my neck, a large set of stickers for whatever car I was using, and reams of papers and instructions saying that I was legitimate. I reported to the deployment area and discovered that the region around Johannesburg and Pretoria had been swamped with thousands of observers. I called a friend at the Independent Electoral Commission office in Cape Town.

"How many observers do you have down there?" I asked.

"Not enough," he said. "Only about three hundred for the entire Western Cape."

I hung up the phone, went outside, hailed a taxi, and went straight to the airport, where I caught a thousand-mile flight to Cape Town. Four hours later I walked into a new set of offices and received a map of where I was to go during the three-day elections. My territory covered the area north and east of Cape Town, including an incredible array of different voting areas: entrenched white Afrikaner towns, destitute African squatter camps, modest Coloured townships, rural plantations where the majority of voters were likely to be illiterate farmworkers.

On Sunday before the election, I called the television station in Boston and asked what the producer wanted me to talk about. He said he wanted me to describe what I had seen as vividly as possible.

"How long do I have?" I asked.

"Two minutes," he replied.

When they started to broadcast, I talked about the people, the preparations, the undercurrent of fear, the pervasive sense of disbelief, and the thousands of police and visitors. At the end the producer came back on the line.

"That was *great*," he said. "Do you think you could do that again?"

"When?"

"How about this time Tuesday and again Thursday?" he said.

"Sure."

And so, much to the consternation of all my competitors and much of the political establishment in Massachusetts, I reported for the next few nights as a foreign correspondent from South Africa. I relished the irony; sitting inside Massachusetts, I had been ignored. When I went overseas, I ended up on television every other night.

As the election day approached, tension mounted. Parties held tumultuous rallies; volunteers attached pictures and slogans to every vertical surface; reporters speculated endlessly on the outcome. Driving along South Africa's most modern highways, I marveled to find the once-banned likeness of Nelson Mandela grinning from the top of every lamppost framed by the words "*MANDELA FOR PRESIDENT*"—thousands of these images, passing rhythmically for miles.

Beneath the fervor of a normal presidential campaign lay a universal sense of amazement, even bewilderment, as people watched the lightning transformation of unattainable fantasies into routine realities. The voting began at seven in the morning on Tuesday, April 26, and stretched over three days. I had persuaded Marijke du Toit, one of my best friends, a female graduate student at the University of Cape Town and daughter of André and Maretha, to join me on this adventure as my driver. Her car was an ancient bright yellow VW bug covered with patches of rust, but we turned it into an official observer car by gluing the bright blue INTERNATIONAL ELEC-

TION OBSERVER signs to each of its door panels. As we drove around the Cape Province and came up on police and military roadblocks, those blue signs caused the officers to step aside and wave us through, sometimes with a crisp salute.

On the first day the voting was limited to the elderly and the infirm, in part to give the officials at each voting site a chance to iron out their procedures. At Groote Schuur Hospital in Cape Town, women in labor and patients who were about to go into surgery insisted on casting their ballots at the hospital's polling site first. At South African consulates and other polling stations around the world, an estimated quarter of a million overseas South Africans began to cast their ballots.

The next morning people began arriving at the polls as early as 4 A.M. Everywhere the lines grew longer and longer. Black and white, young and old, men and women, stood with eagerness and patience, even when the technical arrangements faltered. The autumn rains opened up, and Marijke and I drove from place to place with the windshield wipers operating at a furious pace. Despite these regular soakings, people refused to give up their places in line. In previous years anti-apartheid activists in the huge townships had taken down the street signs in order to make it harder for the police to navigate. We worried that we would not be able to find the polling places, since we often had only the skimpiest address. It turned out to be easy; we would enter a township and make a wide loop through the streets until we came to the end of an incredibly long line. We would then drive along that line—sometimes for a mile, sometimes for two—passing thousands of standing people, until we reached the community building or church that had been designated as the place to vote.

As voters reached the entrance to the polling station, they were greeted by a strange assembly of policemen, foreign observers, peace monitors, party representatives, and IEC officials like us. They moved quickly past a succession of tables. Their identity books were examined and marked with invisible ink, their fingernails checked and then sprayed with long-lasting dye that showed up under ultraviolet light. They were then handed a national ballot and escorted to a standing booth where they could mark their ballots in secret. If they had any difficulties, a throng of officials, including me, would surround them to make sure that the advice they were given was impartial. After depositing their ballots in a sealed box, they collected a second ballot, for provincial government, and voted again. Minutes later they were back outside, their faces bearing a range of emotions from sober dignity to tearstained joy.

In most parts of the country the voting unfolded more smoothly than expected, with fewer crowds, more efficient operations, and, most amazingly, no violence. The polls closed at 7 P.M. on Thursday, April 28. At that very moment I was standing in a small church courtyard in the African township of Langa. Barney Pityana, my lawyer/activist/priest friend, had invited me to go with him to a celebration of the Eucharist at this local church. He had just stepped inside to change into his liturgical robes and I was standing by myself, reliving the magnitude of the last few days. Above me rose the dark and towering impassivity of Table Mountain, which stretched up nearly three thousand feet high. A brilliant white moon shone in a black and cloudless sky. All around me was silence. At the precise moment the polls closed, I began to hear a strange murmuring washing over the high walls of the churchyard. As I listened, I realized that I was hearing people's voices as they came rushing out of their houses. All around me I heard a rising blend of excited conversation, laughter, shouts, and songs. From behind my plaster wall I could not see any people, but as I stood there, I felt emotion sweep through me as well. It was the sound of a nation's soul, rising from the dreams of millions of long-suffering people. A new democracy had been born, and I was hearing the cries of joy at its birth being carried to me on the wind.

CHAPTER EIGHT

Blue AND *Green*

*The gross national product does not allow for the
health of our children, the quality of their education
or the joy of their play. It does not include the beauty
of our poetry or the strength of our marriages, the
intelligence of our public debate or the integrity of
our public officials. It measures neither our wit nor
our courage, neither our wisdom nor our learning,
neither our compassion nor our devotion to our country;
it measures everything, in short, except that which
makes life worthwhile. And it can tell us everything
about America except why we are proud that we are
Americans.*

—ROBERT F. KENNEDY

On April 30, 1994, two days after the South African elections had finished, I stepped off an airplane from Johannesburg in New York. As I made my way through the hallways to the plane to Boston, I stopped at a newsstand to pick up the *Boston Globe*. A few days before I had drafted an op-ed column for the *Globe* and faxed it in the middle of the night. I had no idea if it would run. Opening the newspaper to the editorial pages, I found my piece printed at the top. Titled "Where's the Passion?" the piece contrasted what I had just witnessed in South Africa with the discontent in Massachusetts.

"In Massachusetts hundreds of thousands of adults have become so skeptical of public leaders that they neglect to register, refuse to sign nomination papers, or simply do not bother to vote," I wrote. "We have allowed ourselves to be deterred by inconvenience. This apathy grows from watching one's ideals repeatedly manipulated by others for their personal and political gain. However often we have been disappointed, we must not add to this cycle of cynicism by concluding that the right to vote means nothing." Nowhere had ideals been more grossly betrayed than in South Africa, I pointed out, yet that had driven citizens not to despair but to the ballot box. Their actions raised a question for Massachusetts. "Are South Africans displaying only a rash and youthful hope in democracy," I asked, "or have they shown us how far we have drifted from the enthusiasm and principles on which we built our commonwealth?"

Five weeks later I appeared at the Democratic Party's state nominating convention and discovered that democracy was not completely dead in Massachusetts. In the five minutes I was allotted on the podium, I asked the delegates to give me enough votes to put me on the ballot for lieutenant governor.

To everyone's surprise, I received not only the necessary 15 percent but a decisive 24 percent, even though I had, up to that point, been a complete political unknown. After almost a decade of analyzing, teaching, and writing about social change, as well as witnessing it firsthand on the most profound possible level in South Africa, I had set something important in motion—something that had seemed almost impossible, even foolish, when I began the campaign eight months before.

Over the next four months I rocketed around the state, meeting thousands of people, speaking on topics that moved me, learning the mechanics of elections, defending my views before editorial boards and on television, and working with an exceptional staff and team of volunteers. Eventually I teamed up with a particularly talented driver, Graham Wik, the son of my campaign manager, Lynda. The two of us spent weeks traveling from town to town to town, like two astronauts sent on a distant mission.

I still needed infusions for my hemophilia, so we occasionally had to pull over by the side of the road to do a quick intravenous injection, and we often speculated about how hard it would be to explain to a police officer why I was shooting up. Politically prominent people increasingly returned my calls, so I found myself talking to congressmen and senators and governors, active and retired, about strategy. On one occasion I picked up the phone and the callers were Jimmy and Rosalynn Carter, with whom I had worked years before in New York City on a project for Habitat for Humanity.

"We just wanted you to know that we're both thinking

of you. We believe that you are a wonderful candidate," said Carter.

"Thank you, Mr. President," I said, watching the telephone poles fly by as Graham and I sped down the highway.

Politics is a strange and often wonderful business, I thought as I hung up.

*

As we moved out of the doldrums of summer, I built up steam. Even though my opponent, a hardworking state representative named Marc Draisen, had the official allegiance of 129 of the 130 Democratic state representatives in the State House, I continued to attract support. A month before the primary, a major feature story appeared in *Boston* magazine. Then the *Boston Globe*, the *Boston Herald*, and a host of other newspapers endorsed me. "I wonder if this is what momentum feels like?" I asked Evelyn Murphy, a former lieutenant governor, at one point.

"It is, Bob, it is," she replied.

On primary day I had nothing to do but go to various polling places to greet people, and when even the workers from other campaigns, including Republican ones, wanted to shake my hand, I sensed that I was doing well. That night I won the primary with just under 53 percent of the vote. After fewer than ten months, starting from nowhere, I was now the Democratic nominee for lieutenant governor. I was immediately paired with the winner of the gubernatorial primary, Mark Roosevelt (great-grandson of Theodore Roosevelt), to form the Democratic ticket against the incumbents, Governor Bill Weld and Lieutenant Governor Paul Cellucci.

Weld had no primary opposition and had raised millions of dollars, which he spent ridiculing Roosevelt. I was not even considered worthy of criticism. Weld, it turned out, had a secret agenda; he wanted to win by such a devastatingly large margin that he could take on U.S. senator John Kerry in 1996. To do that, he needed to crush the Roosevelt-Massie ticket.

The White House looked at the race and decided, probably correctly, that with only seven weeks left in the campaign, there was not much that could be done. Nonetheless, President Clinton flew to Massachusetts and spoke on behalf of all the Democratic candidates on a stage in Framingham. I remember arriving early on the stage and seeing pieces of tape on the floor identifying where we should stand. The piece that said "MASSIE" was about eight feet away from a piece of tape that said "POTUS."

"Who's Potus?" I asked a Secret Service man.

He looked at me as if I were a moron. "The *P*resident *O*f *T*he *U*nited *S*tates," he said laconically.

I bounced around the state with national Democrats. I spoke from the same stage as Hillary Clinton in Springfield and was touched to discover that she had read my parents' book *Journey*. I introduced Teddy Kennedy (who was running for reelection against political newcomer Mitt Romney). I learned how to whip up a crowd so that they would greet him with a huge roar as he came chugging up to the stage, with a broad smile and a great slap on the back for me. On one occasion Teddy went out of his way to introduce me. Listening to his resonant baritone talking about this "remarkable young man," I found myself staring at my shoes in disbelief. Finally, just before the election, Vice President Gore flew to Boston to speak at a major fund-raising lunch. This was a special act of friendship, going back to my grandmother's strong support for his father, Al Gore, Sr., during his first Senate race in Tennessee. Though the White House political office counseled against it and Gore was on crutches after tearing an Achilles tendon while playing basketball, the vice president overruled his advisers and came anyway.

All this did not stem the tide, either locally or nationally. The Republican Party had seized on President Clinton's efforts to establish national health insurance and attempted to tear him limb from limb. Newt Gingrich announced his solemn support of the "Contract for America" and got the Republican members of the House of Representatives to line up to sign it. I debated the incumbent Republican lieutenant governor, Paul Cellucci, and learned what it was like to have a political opponent lean within inches of my face when on television to bellow out his answers. Bill Weld kept up his on-air humiliation of Mark.

The night of the election was sobering. I knew that we were going to lose, so I spent a long time preparing my very brief concession speech. We met in the Copley Plaza Hotel, just down the hall from the ballroom where Teddy Kennedy was celebrating his election to a sixth term in the United States Senate. As the numbers rolled, it was clear that we had lost by a large margin: 40 points (70 percent to 30 percent).

To my immense surprise, Rosalynn Carter appeared in person to thank me for my race and to urge me to run again. John Kerry, a long-time friend, came to the room with Teresa Heinz and took me aside. His long face looked worried.

"I'm sorry about your loss," he said. "You did a great job. But this was a super-tough year. The Republicans are winning across the country."

"Did we lose the Senate?" I asked.

"Yes," he said, *"and the House."* That came as a profound surprise and far outweighed my own anticipated loss. He was describing the arrival of what became the 104th Congress, the first House of Representatives controlled by the Republican Party since the 1950s.

When it came time to speak, I delivered my carefully worded critique of the grotesque financial and media carpet-bombing that Bill Weld had inflicted on Mark Roosevelt.

"Just as there is no honor in a mercenary victory," I said, "there is no shame in a principled defeat."

The party ended and I went home.

*

Though I enjoyed myself greatly in politics, the previous few months had been marked by the shock of a completely unexpected action by Dana, to whom I had been married for nearly eleven years. In South Africa we had divided up our time and the care of the children so that we could each make research trips, and she had disappeared for many weekends. She worried more and more intensely that at any moment I would begin my inevitable slide toward AIDS and death. Every cold or cough became in her mind a sign of impending doom. I later learned that at one point, when we both fell ill for several days with a bronchial infection, she was sending secret e-mail messages to my family and friends to say that I was failing and they should prepare for the worst.

We increasingly lived in two worlds, one in which I was happily pursuing my life with my family, whom I loved very much, and the other, in which Dana felt isolated and sorry for me that I was in denial about my fate. At the time there was little in the way of support services for spouses of people with HIV, and our rare efforts to talk about these different experiences of life failed. We stopped trying. I became more outgoing and energetic while she withdrew into a cocoon of loneliness and fear. Eventually she found others from whom she could find support, including someone she came to care about deeply. I knew nothing of all this.

One night in 1994, after my campaign had been well launched, Dana came to me and announced that she had made an irrevocable decision to divorce me. I had no idea that this was coming. My first thought was that somehow she was reacting to the campaign, and I offered to end it instantly, the next day if necessary. She made it clear at that moment and over the following weeks that the campaign had nothing to do with it. Indeed, she said bluntly, she didn't want me around the house trying to persuade her to reconsider. Her decision was final, though she would wait until the campaign was over to announce it. Together we went through many hard months while I did everything I could think of to find another solution. She listened, and she sometimes talked, but from the moment of her announcement she never showed a single sign of changing her mind.

She had been preparing for another life for years, and now she wanted to live it. Her emotional connection to me had been cauterized by my health problems. For years she felt that she had no one to talk to and no one who understood. Originally she had thought that our marriage would end with my death and that she would endure a period of widowhood before moving on. Now, given that I appeared to be so well, the only alternative in her mind was divorce. During the months after the campaign we moved toward this outcome, which finally took place in early 1996. A few weeks after our divorce became final, Dana married the South African professor and missionary whom she had known for more than twelve years.

*

I went back to Harvard Divinity School and started teaching and planning the development of the Project on Business, Values, and the Economy into something bigger and more university-wide. After my experience in politics, my courses focused not just on what should be done but on *how*. It was perfectly acceptable to oppose a company's policies on infant formula or South Africa, I pointed out to my students, but how could you transform that opposition into real improvements? What combination of power and persuasion could be applied to get people to change their minds and their actions?

In approaching these problems I was influenced by the

intensive course on negotiation that I took at Harvard Law School. Taught by the illustrious professor Roger Fisher and a team of talented faculty, the course was built on the groundbreaking insights of Fisher's book with William Ury, *Getting to Yes*. The book revealed the inner structure of most disagreements—for example, that while most people argue about *positions*, they are governed more directly by their unarticulated and underlying *interests*. It swiftly occurred to me that the Divinity School, which tended to focus on the psychological tensions between two people, was missing a major opportunity to talk about how to manage and resolve conflict at the community level. I went back to my dean and proposed that I create a course called "Advocacy, Negotiation, and Reconciliation," which would consist of two hours of theory and two hours of practice every week. He approved it, and suddenly I was teaching the skills that I had only just mastered.

In this course and in all the others I taught I made liberal use of guests from the outside world. During a class on the institutional relationships between churches and corporations, I invited two people to listen to the students make presentations about a particular dispute. One was a senior executive from a major chemical company. The other was Joan Bavaria, the founder of an organization called the Coalition for Environmentally Responsible Economies, or Ceres. Because she lived in the Boston area, she came for lunch beforehand at the Harvard Faculty Club. Within minutes we were fast friends, discussing not only all the points of our common history but all the things we wanted to see happen in the future.

In class, Bavaria did a brilliant job of discussing the challenges of negotiating with large companies about the environment. A few days later she called.

"I don't know how much you know about what Ceres is doing these days," she said, coming straight to the point, "but it has been a board-managed coalition since its inception. We are now ready to bring on a full-time executive director. I would like to sit down with you soon to discuss this job."

Ceres had been formed in 1989 out of discussions among major investment leaders and pension funds on how to apply the lessons of the ongoing South African shareholder campaign to the environment. Ceres had become a powerful force in the aftermath of the *Exxon Valdez* oil spill that devastated Prince William Sound in Alaska; it had originated the definition of an "environmental ethic"—a code of conduct—for corporations modeled in some ways on the Sullivan Principles introduced in South Africa. Ceres had also pioneered the use of an environmental scorecard that asked companies to measure and report their performance against specific goals, and it used a combination of skillful persuasion and raw shareholder power to move companies to make substantial commitments to new environmental and energy plans.

Within a few more months I had made the jump, leaving Harvard Divinity School to become the full-time executive director of Ceres. I was the newest and most senior member of a staff of five, tucked away in cubicles in the back of Joan Bavaria's investment shop. During my first six months, my desk was literally in the stockroom area, so that my phone conversations with foundation program officers and business executives were often interrupted by staff members from the extended company entering the area to get pencils or use the copy machine. I did not even have a computer. I went to work during the day and did my computer work at home at night. To exchange files among our staff, we copied files to a floppy drive and tossed disks over the dividers between our desks.

Despite the modest resources, I realized that I was the head of an unusually broad coalition with enormous potential power. We were the only entity in the United States that brought together the grassroots power of environmental and union groups and the financial clout of major investors and pension funds. Our board and membership were made up of senior representatives of virtually all of America's largest environmental groups: the Sierra Club, the National Wildlife Federation, Friends of the Earth, the World Wildlife Fund, the Union of Concerned Scientists, and many others. We also included pension funds with hundreds of billions in endowment assets, such as those of both New York City and New York State, the Methodist and Presbyterian churches, a large number of Roman Catholic orders and institutions, and the Interfaith Center on Corporate Responsibility. We had a strong tie to labor through the AFL-CIO. Over time the coalition added even more powerful allies, including the California state public employees and teachers funds, along with funds from Connecticut, Maryland, Vermont, and many other denominations and states.

In addition to the unusual alliance between investors and environmental groups, two things made Ceres unique. The first was that we engaged directly with corporations, asking them to commit to an environmental program, measure their performance, and disclose their results. Second, the size and expanse of the funds around the table meant that someone in our network was bound to hold stock in virtually any publicly traded company in America. Thus, for every issue we wanted to discuss we had a very large shareholder who would join us in ringing the doorbell of the company with a request to talk.

Corporations were initially hostile to engaging with us. Their lawyers thought that the firm should maintain maximum independence and combat every potentially encroaching force: state governments, federal regulators, private lawsuits, public-interest groups. When they looked at our ten proposed "Ceres Principles," they saw nothing but trouble. If the principles were in any way binding, they would cause terrible new precedents and problems in the courts. If they were not binding, why go through the exercise of discussing and embracing them?

The principles are worth reprinting here as they appeared in the early 1990s. To some people these sounded like the bare minimum of environmental responsibility, and to others like an aggressive attack on free enterprise.

The Ceres Principles

1) PROTECTION OF THE BIOSPHERE
   We will reduce and make continual progress toward eliminating the release of any substance that may cause

environmental damage to the air, water, or the earth or its inhabitants. We will safeguard all habitats affected by our operations and will protect open spaces and wilderness while preserving biodiversity.

2) SUSTAINABLE USE OF NATURAL RESOURCES
We will make sustainable use of renewable natural resources, such as water, soils, and forests. We will conserve non-renewable natural resources through efficient use and careful planning.

3) REDUCTION AND DISPOSAL OF WASTES
We will reduce and where possible eliminate waste through source reduction and recycling. All waste will be handled and disposed of through safe and responsible methods.

4) ENERGY CONSERVATION
We will conserve energy and improve the energy efficiency of our internal operations and of the goods and services we sell. We will make every effort to use environmentally safe and sustainable energy sources.

5) RISK REDUCTION
We will strive to minimize the environmental, health, and safety risks to our employees and the communities in which we operate through safe technologies, facilities, and operating procedures, and by being prepared for emergencies.

6) SAFE PRODUCTS AND SERVICES
We will reduce and where possible eliminate the use, manufacture, or sale of products and services that cause

environmental damage or health or safety hazards.
We will inform our customers of the environmental
impacts of our products or services and try to correct
unsafe use.

7) ENVIRONMENTAL RESTORATION

We will promptly and responsibly correct conditions
we have caused that endanger health, safety, or the
environment. To the extent feasible, we will redress
injuries we have caused to persons or damage we
have caused to the environment and will restore the
environment.

8) INFORMING THE PUBLIC

We will inform in a timely manner everyone who may be
affected by conditions caused by our company that might
endanger health, safety, or the environment. We will
regularly seek advice and counsel through dialogue with
persons in communities near our facilities. We will not
take any action against employees for reporting dangerous
incidents or conditions to management or to appropriate
authorities.

9) MANAGEMENT COMMITMENT

We will implement these Principles and sustain a
process that ensures that the Board of Directors and
Chief Executive Officer are fully informed about
pertinent environmental issues and are fully responsible
for environmental policy. In selecting our Board of
Directors, we will consider demonstrated environmental
commitment as a factor.

10) AUDITS AND REPORTS

We will conduct an annual self-evaluation of our progress in implementing these Principles. We will support the timely creation of generally accepted environmental audit procedures. We will annually complete the Ceres Report, which will be made available to the public.

Before I had arrived, Joan Bavaria and some of the large shareholders had sat down with a few companies to talk about whether they might endorse the Ceres Principles. Some companies began to move in our direction. Robert Campbell, the CEO of Sunoco, an oil-refining firm, came up to Joan after one meeting and told her that he might be the head of an oil-refining and marketing company, but he shared many of her goals. And he didn't think that there was anything wrong with a company setting targets and trying to meet them. "That's how we do everything else in the firm," he told Bavaria. "We pick a target, we decide how we are going to measure our performance against that target, and then we pursue it. This is pretty much the same."

Joan was delighted to hear this. She had quickly learned that "we manage what we measure" was one of the most powerful mantras in modern business. Two things became clear from this simple phrase. If we could persuade a firm to measure and disclose its performance, we tapped into one of the most powerful internal mechanisms for lasting change within the corporation. However, the reverse was also true: if something was *not* measured, it often was impossible to manage. This fit with everything I had learned since I was a boy about the relationship between sight and sound and words. If a person—or in this case an entire collection of people—had a specific word or measurement that he or she could systematically apply across a vast amount of behavior, then one could both see and change that practice. If not, the actions and consequences were invisible, even to insiders, and especially to anyone outside the organization. So creating change and agreement required developing the ability to imagine how one's apparent opponents saw (or didn't see) parts of the world. Sometimes this meant learning their vocabulary and using it in a way they could understand. Sometimes it meant teaching them a vocabulary that was new to them.

As the board of Ceres realized the power of the idea of measurement, we built our strategy around three steps that we believed could actually move corporate America on to a more environmentally sustainable path. Our process was straightforward. We asked senior executives at a corporation to commit to continuous environmental improvement in partnership with Ceres. Most corporations, in fact, believed in this. What executives fear is abrupt change: a sudden shift in the market, a major disruption in supply or technology, or the random imposition of a new regulation that would change their business model. In the phrase "continuous improvement," we found words that they could embrace.

We then urged them, as a condition of their participation, to set up measurements, following the ten Ceres Principles, to see whether they were making progress. After many years of negotiating with executives I learned that their initial reluctance to take on new challenges is often due not to a lack of energy or courage; instead, they want to take on only those challenges at which they have a reasonable chance of succeeding.

Corporate life is built around selecting a strategy, picking the right indicators, and then aggressively pursuing their targets. One of the problems with integrating the environment was that these ideas had no place in the vast scheme of company strategies, targets, tactics, internal investments, and compensation. If we could graft this new information and these new approaches onto the hugely powerful and effective corporate system for getting things done on an enormous scale, we knew we would have tapped an immense force.

Finally, it was important to ask companies not just to set targets and to measure their performance but to release that information to the public. We assumed that being required to show whether they had improved or slipped would prompt corporate leaders to pursue better results over the years. By releasing the information, the corporation was driving a deeper stake into the ground, not only with outside groups like the activists and investors who made up Ceres but also with the press, with their competitors, and, perhaps most important of all, with their boards of directors and their employees. We also believed that they would gain from the exercise by saving money through eliminating waste, by pushing themselves to innovate into new technologies, by winning new customers and developing new product lines. Environmental improvements also inspired employees, who wanted to believe that they were going to work every day for a reason larger than their own personal paychecks. The positive experience would then strengthen their desire to intensify their efforts and their commitments.

Every negotiation with every company followed its own course. Some jumped on the idea. Some took years to persuade. Some worried that a commitment would mean too much time, energy, and expense. Some thought that they wouldn't really be expected to do very much and could get the public relations benefit of signing without the need for follow-up action. Through dozens of presentations, meetings, and meals, either at Ceres or in conference rooms around the country, we systematically made our case. We reviewed sectors of the economy, chose the most likely corporate participants, and then analyzed each team of executives to understand the arguments they would present and the benefits they could obtain. We asked leaders who had already joined in our effort to speak to those who had not. We acknowledged that some members of the Ceres coalition had different values and objectives from those of these huge firms, but we pointed out why it was to everyone's advantage for us to be in conversation. Over time, more and more executives listened—and signed up.

Through listening to the men and women who represented the companies in our discussions, I realized that though they initially came across as fierce advocates for their corporation's position, they were often relatively weak within their organizations, without the line or budget authority that would give them real clout. Some of the executives we engaged were, ironically, seen as leftist environmental advocates within their own firms. Some of those who argued against us in public were advocating for us in private. Gradually we learned the subtle truth that a person who appears to be an opponent can sometimes be a hidden ally.

*

Measurement and accounting are strange worlds, somewhat like engineering. To outsiders they seem like hopelessly technical and boring fields. To insiders, however, these details determine whether an entire system succeeds or collapses. Much like an engineer knowing the exact degree of lift and thrust necessary to put a massive airliner into the sky, so accounting experts need the specific application of measurement. We realized that even though the technical details might seem obscure, their overall effect could be immense. We learned to speak the corporate language so that we could persuade companies to make adjustments that would alter their interactions with the world. I understood that change was about more than glossy speeches and the affirmation of values, as important as those could often be; it was also about the hard work of proposing the exact, detailed modifications that would cause corporations to behave differently.

After listening to squabbling among different activist and environmental organizations about whose measurement system was best, I asked the heads of ten key groups to meet me at a conference center outside Washington, D.C., to forge a common approach to working with companies. We were spending too much time and energy pointing out small differences between our approaches, I said. There were plenty of times when I appeared before a program officer at a foundation, was asked about all the different proposals for environmental measurement, and found myself saying, "Theirs is good but ours is better." Instead, I suggested, we needed to talk about each other's strengths and find a way to work together. We had to act more like a movement and less like competitors.

In late 1996 and early 1997 I was traveling all around the country as the new head of Ceres, and I asked people what they thought most needed to happen in the field. I spoke to business leaders, environmental activists, investors, academics, and many others. They usually talked about some tactical improvement they wanted to see—a small change in this approach or that questionnaire.

"No, that's not what I'm looking for," I said to dozens of people. "I am asking: What would you like to happen in the field of environmental reporting if you could have *anything*? What is our ultimate goal?"

Business executives said they were tired of being deluged with queries and that they wanted to be able to fill out a single questionnaire that would be accepted by multiple activist groups. Activists, for their part, deeply distrusted the current information that companies released, believing that they would report only on the things that made them look good. And investors pointed to the uselessness of corporate data that could not be compared from company to company.

The disagreements were sharp, but when I asked about the best solution, I discovered to my surprise that there was strong agreement. Every party wanted to develop a single tool for disclosure that would simultaneously meet the needs of executives, activists, and investors. This was, after all, what happened in the financial markets. There had been a time when companies reported their financial results any way they wanted to, but this had contributed to several market collapses. Today companies accept—and the government requires—a single standard. Known as Generally Accepted Accounting Principles (GAAP), these rules allow for measurement and comparison that make sense and thus enable all of American business to function smoothly.

As I listened, an idea became clearer in my head. If creating a standard for finance helped everyone both inside and outside business, why not a standard for measuring all the pieces of sustainability, everything from labor and human rights to energy and the environment? When I suggested this to people, they agreed that this would represent a major advance for business in the world. But no one believed it could happen. There was no group that was willing to lead on this, and governments could never successfully take it on.

*

I have never been inclined to accept the impossibility of a great idea, so I started to plan how we could create what everyone said they wanted. I arranged for a workshop to explore the topic at our next small Ceres annual conference in Chicago in the fall of 1996. The conference went well but the workshop was a bust. To my memory just three people showed up: me, my dear friend and colleague Allen White (a distinguished social scientist at the Tellus Institute), and one other person, who left after it became clear that the workshop was not going to take place.

I was tired after a long day, and I proposed to Allen that we just stay and get a beer in the hotel and use that time to do some forward planning. I told him about the common reaction that I was getting from my queries, and he told me that the research that he was doing on environmental reporting showed that the groups were really not far apart.

"Why don't we just try to do what everyone really wants?" I asked Allen. "People are all saying the same thing, even when they are from very different backgrounds and have very different interests. That ought to give us the starting point to build a new cooperative agreement."

"It's worth a try," said the ever-genial and thoughtful White.

So right then and there we decided to redirect the focus of Ceres, in cooperation with the Tellus Institute, toward developing a common framework for reporting. A key step would be to enlist a steering committee made up of representatives of all the groups who wanted to see the same thing.

To allay people's fears, I set out some principles and rules from the beginning. Ceres would act as an honest broker, with a commitment to include virtually anyone who felt a desire to contribute. We would share information and documents widely on the Internet, which was just starting to become a tool in people's daily work lives. Finally, we committed to spin the new standard-setting body off from Ceres if our efforts succeeded. This last guarantee turned out to be the most critical, because it helped people commit time and resources without the suspicion that they might be handing over a key initiative to a rival.

We struggled with what to call this new project. ITT Industries had pointed out to us that the Ceres questionnaire was very much on U.S. data and U.S. questions. Since ITT was a global company that did more than two-thirds of its business outside the United States, it wanted us to consider developing a "global report" that would apply internationally. My Ceres colleague Judy Kuczewski and I kicked around several names, including "Global Report Initiative," but that seemed too static. We wanted something more dynamic. "Let's try 'Global Reporting Initiative,'" one of us said, and the name stuck. And it quickly became known around the country and around the world by its initials, GRI.

The Ceres board agreed to our plan. I then had to raise the money to do it. Around Easter of 1997 I received a message from a college friend of mine, Ralph Taylor, who had been following my efforts for some time and had briefly participated on the board. In his note he said that he would contribute $80,000 of his own money to get us started and that he wanted me to meet his parents, who could potentially contribute more.

At this time in my life I again could not walk; I had slipped on my back steps at home and badly crushed my left knee, the one I had struggled with as a child. My doctors grimly told me that I would never use that joint again. They recommended a total knee replacement, and in early 1997 they took out the knee and replaced it with an artificial joint made of titanium. For several months I had to run Ceres from my home, using the early technology of e-mail to communicate with my staff, board, and network. I continued to negotiate with the executives of major companies on the phone, though I was grateful that we did not yet have video technology, since I was often in my pajamas with my leg extended in bed. To meet Ralph's parents would require an arduous trip to Florida while the knee was still weak and I was on crutches. I felt the timing was critical, so I went.

I flew to Hobe Sound, one of the wealthiest towns in Florida, and spent two days with Ralph and his family. After twenty-four hours of small talk, his parents took me to their country club for dinner. As we were waiting to be seated, his father, who was sitting across from me on a couch, leaned forward, spun the ice cubes around in his glass, and looked me straight in the eye.

"So you're telling me that if we give you $100,000, you will change the entire system of environmental accounting—and eventually financial accounting—for every business in the world?"

Put that way, the whole idea sounded crazy, especially for such a small sum. But I knew I could not back down.

I fixed my eyes on him. "Yes," I said.

A month later we received the check.

*

One of the early tests of the organization came when Allen White and I went to London so that I could chair an organizing meeting of the GRI in partnership with a key section of the United Nations Environment Programme. The section was headed by a formidable UN division chief, Jacqueline Aloisi de Larderel. We met as the institutional guests of Roger Adams, the director of research for the Association of Certified Chartered Accountants in London. Our meeting took place in a paneled board room with thousand-dollar leather chairs overlooking the spectacular little park called Lincoln's Inn Fields, the home of many of England's most distinguished law firms.

At the meeting one of Europe's greatest visionaries on the relationship between the economy and the environment, John Elkington, wasted no time challenging me and the handful of Americans who had made the trip to state our purpose clearly. In his judgment, the project had to be truly ambitious.

"The United States is generally behind the world on environmental measurement, and we have little confidence that putting our time and effort into such a domestic enterprise would be useful," he said.

I waited for him to continue.

"If, however, you are interested in tackling the whole question of a standard for *sustainability*—that is, taking the environment as a key foundation but also looking at human rights, labor practices, community impacts, and all the other ways that corporations and communities interact—then we believe that this could be very exciting."

I said that this was my intention, and that I would work to win the support of my board. I returned to the United States with a sense of optimism. The logic for building international cooperation was powerful. The United Nations was striving to improve the social impact of businesses in many countries beyond the reach of an American organization like Ceres. At the same time, Ceres had a powerful presence in the United States, the world's largest economy. It was a creative partnership that both sides decided to embrace.

*

The daily demand to solve the problems of logistics and diplomacy required steady and energetic leadership. Sometimes I didn't have time to think. Yet every now and then I was able to pause and consider what we were really trying to do, which was to create a system that would help people and protect the planet. The passion within me was tied to an image that floated in my mind like a dream: a particular photograph of our fragile blue planet hanging in space.

I had first seen it and loved it when the Apollo 17 astronauts returned from the moon in 1970. Their picture showed the earth fully bathed in sunlight from the South Pole. In the late 1980s and early 1990s, I had become aware of the problem of greenhouse gases building up in our atmosphere, slowly creating the invisible blanket of heat-trapping gases that have been steadily distorting the climate of the entire planet. After attending a key meeting in 1991 of some of America's top scientists and religious leaders at the Cathedral of St. John the Divine, I learned more about the dangerous path on which humanity had launched itself. Scientists from around the world were documenting the steady accumulation of greenhouse gases, the resulting rise in average global temperature, the melting of polar ice, and other disturbing trends. Though planetary science is complex, it was clear that allowing human activity to raise the temperature of the planet would lead to more severe weather, including more violent storms, droughts, and floods, which could harm hundreds of millions of people and cost trillions of dollars in property and economic damage.

To make sure that the religious community played an important role, I went to the dean of Harvard Divinity School early in 1991 to ask him to allow me to organize an event in Massachusetts that would enable faculty members from the nine seminaries in the Boston Theological Institute, a cooperative group, to learn more about the climate crisis and to consider how they could integrate these ideas into their curricula. Working with a talented group of graduate students, we secured permission to use the IMAX theater at the Boston Museum of Science, which was showing *The Blue Planet,* a mesmerizing film shot from space by the space shuttle astronauts. My goal was to combine these powerful images with both scientific information and practical reflections about what could be done by the schools. We scheduled the event for April 1992, and we invited Senator Al Gore, who had not yet been chosen for the vice presidential position by Governor Clinton, to come to Boston to speak. We titled the event "The Renewal of Reverence: Theological Education in the Environmental Era." We filled the hall with well over three hundred people.

What has stayed with me ever since are the quiet moments of the evening, as we watched the shuttle fly silently through space and record the aching beauty of Earth. From far above the planet we saw no division of the blue of the atmosphere from the green of our vegetation. Sitting there, I realized that there should be no such divisions in human thinking. Blue might represent labor and green might represent the environmental movement, but we needed to bring them together. Blue might represent the earth and green might represent the economy, but we needed to bring them together. That became my goal and my task.

*

In asking how the Global Reporting Initiative actually got off the ground, people tend to wonder about three things: first, the mechanics; second, the people; and third, the problems that we overcame. Because of the eventual global success of the GRI, these have now been documented by scholars and academic researchers in many languages. As the cofounder and chair for those first years, I can offer a few insights.

First, the mechanics. We conducted an open-source process. Anyone who wanted to be part of the project could participate. The role of Ceres—and then the role of the secretariat, when it emerged—was to help anyone who desired to play a role to do so. Initially that meant that people who were interested in water use and pollution could come together and think about how to measure that. It meant that people who cared about the overall content of a sustainability report could offer their views on that. In the early days, we assigned people who had skills and interests directly to the relevant committees and let them hash out their concerns, without trying to dictate their decisions in any way. We were immensely aided by the sudden rise of the Internet in the late 1990s and the early 2000s. If we had tried to create the GRI just a few years before, it would have been impossible for the far-flung participants to communicate with each other rapidly. Instead, we could hold an in-person meeting, carve out the basic ideas, and then circulate multiple iterations of a draft within weeks—all globally, instantly, and for free. The speed of our success created its own excitement, as people realized that something was really happening and that if they wanted to be involved, they should jump on now.

We also benefited from a marvelous steering committee from many disciplines and parts of the world. At the beginning we had strong representation from Europe and North America. We expanded to bring in representatives of Ford, General Motors, ITT Industries, and Royal Dutch Shell, major environment groups, top international labor officials, senior officials from accounting societies from Europe and Canada, and NGO leaders from Australia, Colombia, Japan, South Africa, India, and other countries.

The reaction I received from one Canadian participant, a nationally recognized leader in accounting, moved me particularly. He came to me and said, "You know, I was starting to reach the end of my career, and I realized that I wanted to be involved, if possible, in one more major effort to change the way the world works. I didn't know if such a possibility would emerge. But I wrote down what I was looking for on a little piece of paper so that if I ever found it, I would remember to be grateful. I have kept that paper in my wallet ever since. Would you like to see it?"

"Yes," I said.

He pulled his wallet out of his pocket and withdrew a sliver of paper. On it he had written, "I want to be involved with a major international effort to rewrite the rules of accounting so that business contributes to the true well-being and sustainability of our beautiful planet." He put the paper away and looked at me with tears in his eyes.

"I wrote this before I had ever heard of you, Bob Massie," he said, "so I thought you might like to know that this whole effort is, in part, the fulfillment of a middle-aged accountant's deepest prayer for his life."

*

We also encountered opposition. While Allen White did a brilliant job as cofounder, wrestling the technical details of the GRI to the ground, my function, particularly as chair of the steering committee, was to keep everyone focused on the same goal and moving productively in the same direction. Many people found the effort disturbing, even shocking, and they were more than happy to inform me of their objections.

Regularly I would be approached by someone with a face that expressed distaste or even anger and who would thrust a finger into my chest.

"I have to tell you, Bob, that this whole enterprise is poorly conceived and is likely to fail."

"Why do you say that?" I would ask, knowing that this is what the person wanted to tell me.

Then the person would launch into a litany of complaints: this was being done wrong, this person had been left out, this other person was a fool who would destroy everything, we should have approached some other group to do some other thing instead—the list was always long and vehemently expressed. The conclusion was always that disaster was imminent. When the person stopped talking, he or she clearly expected me to defend myself. I tried a different approach.

"You know, I think you are probably right," I said. "We may fail. Many of the problems you described are real problems that we need to address, and I don't know if we are going to be able to do it in time."

The person would nod with satisfaction.

"I do know one thing, though," I continued, "which is that it would be less likely to fail if I had your participation in it. You obviously have given considerable thought to what needs to happen. You would be in an excellent position to help us figure out a solution."

The transformation in the person's attitude was often remarkable. Sometimes it came immediately, but usually it took about six months. At that point I would receive an abrupt e-mail: "Bob, I have given what you said a lot of thought, and now I am ready to help."

*

So, over the next three years, we held dozens of meetings all over the world to enlist support. The steering committee made a point of rotating among different cities and institutions, and Allen and I traveled on special road trips that took us to India, Japan, Brazil, South Africa, Kenya, and many other places. We met with business executives, government officials, academics, and NGO leaders. We received millions of dollars in funding from the United Nations Foundation, the MacArthur Foundation, the Ford Foundation, and the General Motors Foundation.

At one point my director of development, Tim Brennan, and I flew to Seattle for a forty-five-minute meeting with a program officer from the Bill and Melinda Gates Foundation to discuss the possibility of a specialized project in which we would measure the prevalence of HIV in southern Africa among workers in labor-intensive industries like sugar and mining. They were interested and asked for a briefing from Allen White, who was leading the research. Allen and I called from separate phones a few days later. Allen brought up the topic of funding.

"Well, I don't know," said the program officer. "For this kind of thing it would have to be a discretionary grant."

I knew Allen was disappointed. Discretionary grants usually amounted to only five to ten thousand dollars.

"How much would that be?" he asked tentatively.

"Well, it would have to be under one million dollars," said the officer apologetically.

I thought I heard Allen stifle a cough on the other end of the line.

In the weeks ahead, we worked up a budget for $970,000 that would allow us to do a top-notch job. We sent off the proposal with great uncertainty. Three days before the 9/11 terrorist attacks a plain envelope arrived in the regular mail. I opened the letter and out fell a check for the full amount.

During this period various working groups were busy designing the guidelines. To demonstrate the clear compatibility of our effort with financial accounting, we worked with accounting experts to adopt the core principles of transparency, inclusiveness, auditability, and completeness. Differences in language and perspective required a delicate and careful hand. At one point relatively early in the process, I urged that the GRI commit to a certain "form" that would enable people to understand how the information was being collected and used. Roger Adams from England objected vehemently. The GRI did not need a form, he said. I continued: but how could the GRI function if we did not give it a particular structure?

"I'm all for structure," he said. "I just don't think that the GRI should have a form."

A light bulb went off in my head. "What do you mean by the word '*form*'?" I asked.

"You know—a form, a *questionnaire*," he said testily.

I laughed. I realized that though we were both English-speakers, we had stumbled on the different meanings of the same word. "'*Form*' does not automatically mean 'questionnaire' in American English," I told Roger.

"Well, it does where I am from!" he said.

*

After several years it became clear that the original experiment to see whether organizations from around the world could be drawn into working on a common measurement for sustainability had been a success. The question then became whether it was now time to spin off the organization from Ceres into an independent group with a completely new board. We made the decision to "institutionalize" at a key meeting with board members and funders in Toronto in 2000, and within two years we had met that goal as well.

On April 4, 2002, hundreds of people assembled from around the world at United Nations headquarters in New York to celebrate the inauguration of the GRI as a permanent standard-setting body. To create a strong wind at its back, we had assembled a "charter group" of twenty-six international organizations, including huge activist organizations such as Amnesty International, Human Rights Watch, Greenpeace, and the World Conservation Union, to participate. We also had the support of the United Nations, a host of global corporations, and major accounting and sustainability organizations everywhere. Leaders from around the world sent their best wishes and expressions of support. "Companies that win the public's confidence and trust are open, visible, engaging, and create business value while delivering benefits to society and the environment," wrote Bill Ford, the chairman of Ford Motor Company. "The Global Reporting Initiative guidelines . . . provide the disclosure framework that businesses need to report fully on their economic, environmental, and social performance."

As I stood before the group that morning in the delegates' dining room at the UN, I found it hard to get a grip on my emotions. In less than four years, we had taken an idea that seemed completely unreasonable and created a powerful new body that was already transforming the world economy. The guidelines had been translated into eight languages and were in use by hundreds of corporations; they were well on the way to becoming the standard for global measurement and performance.

Along with Timothy Wirth, the president of the United Nations Foundation, and the head of the United Nations Environment Programme, Klaus Töpfer, I was one of the main speakers. I started with a reference to the biblical story of the mustard seed, in which something impossibly small at the beginning grows into something impressively large at the end. How did that happen? I asked. "It grew whenever an individual human being decided to participate, to contribute something," I told the group. "Every decision by every person to add an idea, to offer assistance, to articulate a critique in the spirit of improvement, helped it to grow."

At the same time, this was still an inauguration, a beginning. We had started something important, but we were not finished. The challenges that we faced in the world were bigger than any one country or part of society; they reflected a challenge to our whole industrial civilization, as we attempted to create prosperity for the people without damaging the planet. I quoted a portion of a beautiful poem by Gerard Manley Hopkins:

Generations have trod, have trod, have trod;
And all is seared with trade; bleared, smeared with toil;

And wears man's smudge and shares man's smell: the soil
Is bare now, nor can foot feel, being shod.

And for all this, nature is never spent;
There lives the dearest freshness deep down things . . .

We had engaged in the effort to create the GRI, I said, because even though we understood the value of work and growth and prosperity, we did not want to live in a world known only for being seared with trade and smeared with toil. We wanted to believe that human dignity and earthly beauty could also be protected and enhanced. "We have been bold," I concluded, "but we must be bolder still."

I stepped down from the podium—and thus from the chair of the first board—to an ovation, and I knew that one major piece of my life had just come to an end. I just didn't realize how conclusive that end truly was or how hard would be the new challenges I was about to face.

CHAPTER NINE

Life AND *Death*

The night before the launch of the Global Reporting Initiative I stayed in a small hotel a few blocks from UN headquarters. The Ceres team ran to the building early the next day to make preparations, and I had the chance to walk over alone, enjoying the sunshine and light breeze of an April morning. Even though the distance was only a few blocks, the trip was not easy. My left knee replacement had worked well, but now, nearly four years later, my right knee had degenerated into a painful joint. Bone scraped on bone, causing me to wince with every step. It was obvious that the right knee was also going to have to be operated on. I had traveled around the world with constant pain, waiting until we had completed the task of setting up the GRI, but now the surgery loomed, in less than six weeks.

I was also tired—more tired than I should have been. It had been demanding to run two organizations at once—to serve as the chief executive of Ceres and the chair of the GRI steering committee at the same time. It meant that in addition to making all the daily decisions, I was leading a board meeting in some capacity every six weeks, usually in different cities. I was fortunate that Allen White had taken over the interim CEO position for GRI and moved to Amsterdam to make sure that events ran smoothly there, but I was still responsible for much of the large-scale design and diplomacy of the new institution. Over time the cumulative effect of the travel and the responsibility had started to wear me down, but I sensed that something potentially more serious was wrong with me. When the ceremony at the United Nations ended, I was once again exhausted, and I knew that it was time for another round of tests.

*

Often, even though life can be terribly painful, one is blessed with a moment of mercy. Eight years before, I had been struggling with the shock of having lost my marriage, but soon afterward something unexpected and totally wonderful happened: I reconnected with a woman whom I had known very slightly in college. Anne Tate was a brilliant, beautiful, redheaded architect. We had many friends in common, and she had supported me during the campaign. When it became clear that Dana was never going to change her mind, Anne and I started to spend more time together. Within months I had fallen deeply in love with her, and after a year of courting, she agreed to marry me. We were engaged in 1995 and married in June 1996, and she has been the source of most of my happiness ever since.

Since the issue of HIV had been so destructive in my first marriage, I decided to present myself to doctors in the Boston area to ask them if they had any idea why I was still healthy. By testing frozen samples of my blood that they maintained for routine federal studies, they established conclusively that I had been infected in 1978. I realized with a shock that the mysterious illness that had forced me to withdraw from Yale Divinity School had, in fact, been the acute symptoms of initial HIV infection. Now, seventeen years later, I seemed to be brazenly defying the odds. Eventually I met Dr. Bruce Walker, an infectious disease scientist at Massachusetts General Hospital. "I had my doubts at first about whether he was really infected," he explained to a reporter several years later, "but we confirmed that very quickly and discovered that his viral load was below the limits of detection. That went against what we thought HIV did. It made us extremely interested in learning how he was able to succeed in combating this while others were clearly failing."

In most HIV patients, he explained, cells that fight infection—"the infantry," as he referred to them—are present, but they are missing the "general" cells that tell the infantry what to do. The lack of a coordinated defense opens up the human body to attack by the HIV virus, which can then overwhelm the immune system. When the doctors tested my blood, they expected to find a depleted system of generals. Instead they found enormous numbers of them. They had never seen anything like this, and according to Dr. Walker, it "fundamentally changed how the entire field looked at HIV." "For me it was the first indication that the immune system might actually be able to get the upper hand against HIV," Walker told the reporter. "He's really the person who allowed for that discovery to happen."

Soon Walker was drawing my blood on a regular basis; sometimes he even stopped by our house himself early in the morning to draw it while we drank coffee and talked about the emerging science. Eventually his laboratory shipped samples of my blood all over the world under the research code name 161J. Walker and his colleague Dr. Eric Rosenberg became my very close friends, and they both joked that I could not leave the Boston area without jeopardizing their supply of blood from what they increasingly referred to as "their gold standard."

Ever since then Bruce Walker and his army of grad students have been exploring every aspect of my biochemistry and genetics. Once I was introduced to a large group of Bruce's students at a party at his house. They didn't recognize my name, but when they learned that I was 161J, they flocked around me as if I were a minor rock star. As more and more years passed after my infection—twenty years, twenty-five years, thirty years—it became clear that I was one of the extremely rare people (fewer than one in five hundred) who have a natural genetic resistance to HIV. My unusual situation has prompted several national documentaries, including a prizewinning film for the science program *Nova* in 1998. The information gathered by Dr. Walker, Dr. Rosenberg, and many others over the years gradually gave Anne and me the confidence to try to have a child. On June 18, 1998, our daughter, Katherine Suzanne Tate Massie, was born—a healthy and beautiful girl who has the outgoing temperament of her father and the quick intelligence and fiery hair of her mother. After all the anxiety that my infection generated in my first wife, my family, and my friends, it turned out in the end that even though I had been infected for more than thirty years, I had remained immune to HIV.

The story is still unfolding. Just recently Dr. Walker and an extended national team of researchers decoded the precise genetic sequences of a sample of people like me, and discovered that our resistance came from a specific sequence of amino acids, further opening the door to understanding and treatment. The exact mechanism through which this genetic variation prevents HIV infection, however, remains unknown.

*

By the time of the Global Reporting Initiative event at the United Nations, Kate was three years old and I was traveling extensively to promote the new organization in countries all over the world. The rising knee pain and general fatigue did not bode well. Dr. Walker and then eventually Dr. Raymond Chung at Mass General studied this more carefully and learned that though I had a strong resistance to HIV, another virus, hepatitis C, was causing serious damage. Hepatitis is a slow-moving infection which I had also received through my injections of blood products—yet another illness that could have been avoided if the pharmaceutical companies had heat-treated their products back in the 1970s. Hepatitis attacks the liver over years, even decades. As the liver becomes inflamed, the disturbed cells start making scar tissue, and the organ becomes increasingly gummed up and dysfunctional. The process is irreversible. As this condition, known as cirrhosis, advances, the liver loses its ability to cleanse the blood and create new, critical proteins. Slowly but steadily a person with cirrhosis loses the energy to function.

I had the knee replacement surgery in June, but I had terrible trouble recovering from it. I had planned to travel back to South Africa in August to speak at the World Summit on Sustainable Development, but as I approached the date of departure, I knew that I was in trouble. With deep regret—and not a little foreboding—I canceled that critical trip and took myself into Mass General yet again.

I told Dr. Chung that I was sinking into fatigue. I could not recover from airplane trips. I was beginning to lose focus in the middle of the day. Ray decided to do a full battery of tests. He promised to call me as soon as he had the results.

I was walking across the Boston Common on a beautiful early evening in the fall of 2002. The fading sunlight illuminated the red and amber leaves in the park and made the golden roof of the State House glow. The sight made me realize once again why I love Massachusetts. Then the phone in my pocket buzzed.

"Bob, this is Ray," the doctor said. "Your tests are back. Things don't look good. You are developing advanced cirrhosis, and we recommend that you begin a course of treatment immediately. I need you to come in tomorrow."

I hung up. The evening light had suddenly darkened.

When I went in, Dr. Chung explained that the treatment, which consisted of weekly injections of interferon, would be difficult. It would take four months to see if the treatment was working, and then I would have to continue for a year if it showed promise. The statistics indicated that for my genotype the likelihood of success was small. But we needed to try.

And what would this mean for my work? I asked.

"You may be able to continue, but at a much slower pace," he said. "People react differently. You could be seriously incapacitated."

Within a few months I could barely function. The combination of the cirrhosis and the interferon felt like pianos dropping on me from the sky. In January 2003, I called together the board and staff of Ceres. Since my condition would inevitably deteriorate, the longer I waited, the more I risked the future of Ceres. With a sense of great emptiness and loss, I resigned.

I immediately went home to a largely silent house. A few weeks before I had been traveling the world, guiding and managing two large staffs, giving speeches, orchestrating change, and then everything stopped. Except for seeing a small circle formed by my wife and children and a few friends and caregivers, I had to withdraw into long days of isolation, much as I had for many years as a child in braces and in my wheelchair. I felt as though I had been fired—by life. The possible solution was a liver transplant, but that lay far in the future. No one knew how long the wait would be, or whether the surgery would ever happen at all. If I developed a serious infection or liver cancer, or if the doctors never found an appropriate match, I would die in the next few years.

For the first months I was lost in grief. Hemophilia had been painful and dangerous. HIV had seemed fatal. I had beaten both of those. Now I was facing a new, equally challenging foe, one that I had no guarantee of defeating. I had no sense of the timing, because I was not yet sick enough to qualify for a transplant. When I told my friend and pastor, Michael Povey, that I would have to get much worse before I would rise on the list and qualify for a transplant, he said with compassion (and a touch of humor), "My gosh, Bob, then what do we pray for?"

More than once during those first days I thought of all the biblical characters who had to endure long periods of physical or emotional trial—Job, sitting in ashes; Jonah, lying in the belly of the whale; Moses, wandering for decades toward the Holy Land; and Jesus, stranded in the desert. There is no glamour to waiting; all the excitement of modern life is built around being busy, which is equated with being important. For years I had had responsibilities, opportunities, friends, challenges—and now everything except my wonderful family had been wiped away. I was sitting at home with little to do. I felt as though I had a severe flu—all day long, every day, month after month. I often recalled the words of Paul, who cried out in his letter to the Romans, "Wretched man that I am! Who can deliver me from this body of death?"

For the first year I tried to stay busy and to bring new ideas into being. In the months before I stepped down, I had flown to San Francisco to perform the wedding of Kelsey Wirth, the daughter of Tim and Wren Wirth, all dear friends. On the morning after the ceremony I had collared Tim in the lobby of the Fairmont Hotel and asked him to sit with me for an hour while I explained my latest idea to him. I had realized that Congress was unlikely to take the issue of climate change seriously for years to come, and I had imagined different ways in which to increase the power of investors on this question. Now that the Global Reporting Initiative had been established, I wanted to shift the entire focus of Ceres to the impact of sustainability—and particularly climate change— on the long-term financial value of major pension funds. I proposed to Tim that he help me create an "institutional investor summit on *climate risk*" (a new term) at the United Nations. The idea seemed simple. We would form a group of prominent "conveners" who would invite state treasurers and other pension trustees—who control hundreds of billions of dollars— to the United Nations for a briefing on the long-term effect of climate change on their portfolios. Tim and I, having been in politics, knew that under the right circumstances, state treasurers might jump at the chance to go to New York and think about their special duties as elected representatives responsible for the future of their investment funds and the future of the planet. The venue—one of the major chambers at the UN—would encourage them to take the broad, international, long-term view. The UN, I hoped, would be pleased to have representatives with so much money concentrating attention on one of their signature issues. And then, having gathered the trustees to the UN, we would invite the actual asset managers—the people who controlled the investments on behalf of the treasurers and pension funds—to come listen to something that they were reluctant to consider.

Tim agreed to begin implementing this idea immediately. It took almost a year, and it was not easy. The UN turned out to be skeptical about inviting these "local officials"—it was used to dealing with heads of state. The treasurers were cautious about being associated with the UN, which was under attack by the administration of George W. Bush for being a dangerous, anti-American institution. And the asset managers, who generally believe that if a topic is important, they already know everything there is to know about it, were reluctant at first to come to the UN.

We persisted, however, and eventually sent out an invitation with five pages of signatures from the heads of major organizations asking people to come. Though I was no longer the head of Ceres, my successor, Mindy Lubber, asked me to write some of the speeches for the people who appeared, including Leon Panetta, the former White House chief of staff, who would make the case that the problems were urgent. "The question that every manager or trustee needs to ask is simple," I wrote into Panetta's remarks. *"Under what circumstances and to what degree would our portfolio be affected by climate change?"* To underscore the point, he repeated it.

The event was a huge success, attracting hundreds of the top financial managers to the United Nations and creating a large new force on Wall Street to consider the effect of climate change. Ceres transformed this initial gathering into a powerful organizing tool known as the "Investor Network on Climate Risk," which eventually brought together one hundred members with more than $10 trillion in assets to consider the question and to invest money in clean energy. There have now been four more investor summits. A few months after I stepped down, the Skoll Foundation presented Ceres with the prestigious national Skoll Award for Social Entrepreneurship, which Mindy Lubber accepted on the organization's behalf.

*

At home I struggled to keep going with projects that engaged the outside world. Over the next few years I tried my hand at putting together an Internet company with the modest goal of providing education for everyone everywhere in the world for free. I went so far as to draft a business plan and make presentations to a few prominent venture capital firms in Boston, but my fading energy remained an understandable concern for all of them. Anne and I worked intermittently on various political campaigns, holding one of the earliest major house parties in our region for a candidate for governor, Deval Patrick, who became a friend and went on to win the race. Patrick fully justified our early enthusiasm, except on the issue of gambling, when he entertained a proposal to open up casinos and slot barns all over the state. I examined the matter closely and realized that even though the governor, the senate president, the speaker of the house, and all the major unions (including the teachers' union, which shocked me) were supporting this idea, it would be catastrophic for the poorer people in the state. Working with a wonderful team of allies from across the commonwealth, we attacked slot machines as particularly dangerous because they are designed to create neurological addiction. The best I could do, however, was to attend a few meetings and, on two occasions when I felt physically horrible, drag myself up to the State House to testify against the proposals. We were able to hold the line for several years—and even to adjust the governor's thinking a bit—but the tens of millions of dollars of special-interest casino money, combined with the dazzled but wrongheaded thinking on the part of revenue-desperate legislators and building-trade unions hammered by unemployment, have since carried the day.

I also worked on energy efficiency, bringing together many different parties to promote the adoption of insulation and better technologies for the one million leaky oil-heated homes in Massachusetts where families are struggling to make ends meet. As I had in other settings, I discovered that many people with common interests—from the people who worked with inner-city youth on building rehabilitation, to the low-income fuel assistance advocates, to the clean technology entrepreneurs, to social justice activists, to the energy auditing and retrofit companies, and many others—didn't know each other. When I brought them together, they found common cause and presented a string of proposals to the governor and the legislature. At one point I wrote a piece for the *Globe* in which I argued how the simple act of improving the fuel efficiency of a home would have five positive effects: 1) increasing disposable income by lowering costs ; 2) improving housing values; 3) creating local jobs; 4) advancing the adoption of new technology; and 5) benefiting the low-carbon economy as part of the battle against climate change. The *Globe* ran the story and the new coalition made serious strides, including being part of the effort to persuade the Obama administration to adopt what became known as the "Cash for Caulkers" program. But quickly I had to slip away.

Such engagements were sporadic, demanding, and brief. Mostly I sat at home, trying to balance my intense desire to be engaged with the world with my declining energy. The symptoms of liver disease slowly affected not only my body but also my thinking. The physical fatigue was causing me to sleep twelve, fourteen, even sixteen hours a day. When I was awake, my brain often seemed in a fog. As I explained to one person who came by to write a story for Princeton, "You go through a period where everything slows down. You're still completely awake, but you can't think about things as quickly." I sometimes couldn't think if two people were talking in the room at the same time. I regularly closed my eyes in order to focus on the next words I wanted to say. Concerned that my reaction time was slipping, I completely stopped driving, which meant that I had to rely on Anne, on friends, and on taxis to keep any appointments or leave the house.

With thousands of hours ahead of me and nothing to do, the Internet became my window to the world, and I traveled across it with endless fascination. I set goals for myself. I watched dozens of movies, putting myself through my own version of film school. I learned to make pie crust and turned the sour cherries that grew on the corner of Sycamore and Browning streets into memorable desserts. I also decided to read a biography of every president of the United States. I learned just how often the United States has been in crisis, and how vociferously political opponents have been attacking each other since the beginning of the Republic. I learned hundreds of interesting details—for instance, that George Washington disliked Thomas Jefferson, that Jefferson opposed the creation of an American navy, and that Jefferson and Adams battled bitterly over our relationship with France and England, eventually reconciling twenty-five years after the Declaration of Independence. I learned about the furious arguments over the Mexican-American War, including a passionate speech in opposition by Abraham Lincoln during his sole term as a congressman, and how many of its veterans later became president. I felt unexpected sympathy for the more obscure presidents, including Franklin Pierce, who lost all three of his children before he became president and whose eleven-year-old son died in front of him in a train accident only weeks before his inauguration, an event he tried to drown in alcohol during most of his presidency. (He eventually died of cirrhosis.)

I learned how the politics of the United States never stopped evolving, so that leaders like Martin van Buren, who was a northern Democrat, and John Tyler, who was a southern Whig, eventually found themselves without followers and without parties. Tyler was an especially peculiar president, a man who fathered fifteen children in two sets, starting in 1815 and stretching until 1860. Tyler refused to talk about the "nation" of the United States, because the only nation to which he felt loyalty was Virginia.

I learned how political parties gradually shifted views. I found the Republican Party under Lincoln attractive for its antislavery views and was even more compelled by the Radical Republicans, who fought for the rights of African-Americans during the presidency of Andrew Johnson. I learned with dismay about the rampant racism of the southern Democratic Party, sentiments that endured into the years of my childhood. I noticed how our greatest presidents had certain skills in common. They often combined a clear vision with a canny sense of how to seize unexpected events to advance their purpose in the face of strong opposition.

As my liver slowly collapsed, I slept more and more—sometimes as much as twenty hours a day. Much of the daily burden fell on Anne, who kept working as a professor at the Rhode Island School of Design, took me to medical appointments, cooked meals, and raised Katie. A circle of friends from all parts of our lives, including members of our families and the community of St. James's Episcopal Church in Cambridge, stepped in to support us. As I became disturbingly gaunt and my skin took on an unpleasant grey and yellow hue, they overcame their worry and embraced me. They brought casseroles and treats, drove me wherever I needed to go, and helped to sustain the household. Others banded together to set up an emergency fund for our rising and potentially catastrophic medical expenses. To make sure that I was properly fed, did not have any accidents, and withstood the long empty hours, some individuals committed to staying in our home while Anne was at work and Katie was at school. During birthdays and holidays the members of my family labored mightily to create a festive setting while I dozed on the couch. Looking back, much of this time has faded for me into the haze of partial memory, but for Anne and for our friends it was an intense marathon of care that lasted for years.

Because my condition was deteriorating slowly, there came a point when the only medical option that might rescue me would be to pursue a "living donor" transplant. In this procedure a donor contributes a portion of his or her own liver, which would have been transferred into me. This is feasible because the liver has the extraordinary ability to regenerate, so the separated segments would have grown back to full size in a few months. Because this was major surgery, we doubted that anyone would even consider it; yet when our physicians held the first informational meeting at the hospital, more than a dozen astonishingly generous people came to explore the idea. When the need for a living donor was shared through the Princeton network and on our own Web page, more potential volunteers from around the country stepped forward. Several people went through preliminary testing. One dear friend even received initial approval until, just six weeks before the scheduled surgery, the surgeons abruptly ruled him out because of differences in the anatomy of our veins.

The snow and the flowers and the heat of summer all came and left and came back and left again, year after year after year. My children grew. My friends took new and interesting jobs. As the weeks became months and the months became years, Anne stood as a heroine of stability and compassion. When I lost heart, she encouraged me. My only job, she told me as we talked at night, was to keep going. I could measure the passage of months by watching the top branches of the sycamore tree outside my bedroom window grow; over the years, I saw the leaves reach, surpass, and then conceal the phone wires across the street.

I had no idea where or when it would end. I longed to be back out in the world, meeting people, creating change. At first I was like a racehorse locked in a barn, staring wistfully at the huge fields in the distance. Eventually I dwindled into a weakened creature who was almost constantly asleep.

My medical condition was not promising. My model for end-stage liver disease (MELD) score stayed stubbornly in the middle range, meaning that I was not moving higher on the transplant list. Eventually my Mass General team encouraged me to be cross-listed at another transplant center, and we explored several, including Emory University in Atlanta. It took hundreds of hours to manage all the medical, practical, and insurance details of my care, leading us to wonder how people with fewer resources or a smaller network could possibly cope.

Starting in 2007 I slipped more and began to receive calls for transplants, as either the primary or the backup recipient. Eleven times the phone rang. Each time my family prepared a bag, I stopped eating and drinking for twelve hours, and we nervously held on to our cell phones. Once, on a beautiful spring morning that was also opening day for the Red Sox at Fenway Park, I was told that a jet was warming up on a runway in Cleveland, ready to fetch me. The mayor of Somerville, Joe Curtatone, graciously arranged for me to be taken to the airport in a police car if that proved necessary to get through the baseball traffic. Anne rushed home from RISD, desperately calling people on her cell phone, while Katie, who was only nine, packed her mother's clothes. Then the doctors told the pilots to stand down; it was a false alarm. Twice I made it into Mass General and was prepped for surgery, only to have the surgeons reject the donor organ and send me home.

Over six and a half years Anne and I visited four transplant centers, in Boston, Cleveland, Atlanta, and Pittsburgh, and I was listed in the first three. Each center had its own protocols and tests. We sat forever in windowless beige rooms with old magazines and forlorn fish tanks, waiting for me to be scanned, poked, and prodded in endless tests, consulting legions of physicians, filling out the same medical histories over and over again, and picking through dreary cafeteria food between appointments. As the months dragged by, I felt trapped in the same medical cage that had dominated my childhood. Everyone was pleasant and professional, but I was losing hope.

Finally, in June 2009, I was sitting in my home when the Emory transplant team in Atlanta called with an extraordinary proposal. They had just learned about a twenty-four-year-old patient from Florida who had been living for many years with Maple Syrup Urine Disease, a condition in which she lacked a critical enzyme that processed protein. She had been on a tightly restricted diet since birth. Now, as an adult, she was being exposed to greater and greater risk of brain damage and death. If she received a new liver, her enzyme levels would be boosted enough to process protein and save her life.

The surgeons at Emory realized that when they removed her liver, they would have a young organ that was healthy except for the enzyme problem. If her liver was placed in someone else, through a so-called "domino transplant," the recipient would experience a very slight drop in the enzyme level, but not enough to replicate the young woman's condition. In their view, I was the right match. Anne and I talked to many doctors about whether the solution made medical sense, and they all said yes. When we agreed to the procedure, the team at Emory asked us to come to Atlanta soon.

Our whole family swung into gear to support us. We first drove Katie, now eleven, to Maine so that she could stay for an extended period with our families; we knew that it might be weeks or months before we saw her again. As soon as we arrived, we received a second call from Atlanta: please come now. We threw everything back into the car, kissed Katie goodbye, and drove late into the night to reach Boston. Early the next morning we flew south.

When we arrived, we moved into a special residential facility for transplant patients and their families. We met people waiting for hearts and lungs and livers, and people recovering from their surgeries. We had been there for a week when the transplant coordinator called after midnight. *Please come in at 2:30 in the morning,* she said. Anne and I shook ourselves awake, and then, with nothing to do, we decided that I needed a haircut. We sat in the kitchen under the fluorescent lights, surrounded by newspapers on the floor, while Anne trimmed my unruly hair. Then, in the pitch dark, we drove through the silent streets to the hospital.

The full preparation took nearly twenty-four hours. Anne's sister and her husband drove in from another city to keep us company. Anne also took her computer and issued bulletins on Facebook. Hundreds of people followed our situation and sent good wishes, which she immediately passed along to me. Eventually the chief surgeon, Dr. Stuart Knechtle, brought in the surgeons who would be operating in two teams in side-by-side operating rooms. They stood around my bed in their white coats, lit from above, all of them grinning. To me they looked like angels. When I was introduced to the surgeon who was actually going to be operating on me, Dr. Winston Hewitt, I saw instantly that he was a Jedi knight. He exuded such calm and competence that something within me completely and permanently relaxed.

Late the next night Anne and I were finally called down into the presurgical area. I lay on my back in a room with a dozen empty beds, in my surgical gown, with all my IVs running and Anne at my side. I felt like an astronaut before a launch. My mind skidded through a hundred thoughts and feelings. When I broke free from the atmosphere of my current life, what would I find? Where would I go? Would I ever see this woman sitting beside me again?

Anne pulled out an iPod and we each put in one of the earphones. A few months before, one of our friends had recorded singing in our church, and we now turned to these ancient songs, sung by many of our closest friends, to comfort us. One of the most beautiful is a South African call-and-response setting of the Nicene Creed called "Nasadiki," which means "I believe." The song, led by our dear friend Tom Hirschi, filled our ears with harmony and peace as we waited in a freezing, empty, high-tech waiting area, buried somewhere in a building in Georgia, surrounded by the blues and whites of medical equipment and the quiet and dark of the early morning hours.

The song in the night reached into the deepest part of my soul and reassured me that in the end, I had nothing to worry about. Tom's soaring voice reminded me that out past those walls, there was always going to be a beautiful world, and that out past that world, there was always going to be a glorious universe, and that out past that universe, there was an overwhelming love at the root of everything that would catch me if I fell.

Then members of the operating team came to get me, and with great tenderness Anne kissed me and said goodbye. They took me into an ice-cold, brilliantly lit room, where I was surrounded by bustling people in caps and masks. They moved me onto the operating table, gently positioned my arms and legs, and spoke to me quietly. And then, as it says in the Gospel of Luke, I launched out into the deep, delivering myself wholeheartedly into the hands of others and into an unthinking darkness from which I had no idea if I would ever return.

*

For a long time everything was blackness, emptiness, until slowly it wasn't, and I began to hear voices and feel people moving my body and painlessly removing the tubes that had kept me alive. I recovered consciousness and found myself in intensive care, with Anne, looking tired but relieved, standing beside me. The nurses bustled around and offered quiet encouragement. The doctors came in and spoke to me, and their voices seemed to come from a long way off.

As the hours and days passed, I returned to this life. My recovery during the first weeks was hard—the medical staff watched every heartbeat, every breath, and every change in my body chemistry with vigilance. I experienced strange and difficult symptoms—flashes of intense cold, sudden exhaustion and sweating, accumulation of fluid in my abdomen—but they addressed each one. The nurses, who came from around the world but all spoke in southern accents, took care of me with skill, affection, and good humor. My sister Susanna traveled from her home in Kentucky to make sure I was okay.

After a week of recuperation, Dr. Knechtle approached me with an interesting request: Did I want to meet my liver donor? Anne had already guessed that the donor was somewhere on the same floor, and she even had an idea of who it might be, but this was a direct invitation to meet. I said that I would be delighted to do so, if she was also willing. The word came back that she was. At the appointed moment we gathered—the two families, several doctors, a few nurses and social workers.

Dr. Knechtle suggested that we start by talking about our lives before transplantation and what it meant to us that we had gone through the procedure. I learned that my donor, a charming young woman named Jean Handler, had lived with her illness and its frightening implications from the moment of her birth. She had been forced to eat a rigorous and highly tedious diet; she had never tasted anything with a significant amount of protein until the days after the surgery. I talked to her about what it was like to grow up with hemophilia. I mentioned the joint bleedings, the pain, and the long stretches of isolation and missed school. At different moments during our presentations, everyone in the room choked up and we had to pause for a second before we could go on.

We chatted more and more comfortably about the details of life in the aftermath of transplant. We both knew that we had a long recuperation in front of us. Jean told me about tasting ice cream and meat and other previously forbidden foods for the first time. We agreed that the nursing staff was the best we had ever known. Eventually we started to tire, so we decided to meet again in a few days.

As we got ready to depart, I leaned forward and concentrated my attention on Jean.

"Jean, I just want to express my gratitude as deeply as I can. This was an extraordinary act of generosity on your part. It is going to change my life completely."

She let out a light and breezy laugh.

"Oh, Bob, of course!" she said with a huge smile. "Any time!"

*

In those first weeks and months of recuperation, the doctors focused on the critical issue of whether my body would accept the foreign tissue of Jean's liver. They measured and adjusted my anti-rejection drugs daily. They also wanted to be sure that by suppressing part of my immune system they did not cause the HIV and hepatitis viruses to get out of control, so they put me on medications to control those. For eight weeks I continued living at the transplant house, struggling with the many complicated symptoms that emerge in the first few months of a new organ. Again Anne took care of me as I mastered the new medications and overcame each challenge. Katie came for a visit, and it was a thrill to see her, though she struggled with her disappointment that I was not "all better yet." Soon it was time for us to go home and begin our new life.

When we finally packed up and left for the airport, I experienced a moment of disorientation. All our bags were ready, but I could not find the "shot bag" in which I carried the material for my hemophilia. I instinctively looked for it. Then I was reminded of the truth: Jean's liver, residing in me, was now successfully churning out Factor VIII at normal levels. I did not need the shot bag—and I never would again, for the rest of my life.

I sat down on the bed and put my head in my hands, overwhelmed with emotion. Sitting there in that little room, I realized that the deepest and most secret desire of my childhood, the dream of the crippled Superman, the desperate cry of the boy suffering through the brutal joint bleedings that kept me from walking and from sleep, had finally been heard. In addition to my salvation from HIV and from hepatitis C, I had experienced a miracle that stretched all the way back to my first flickering thoughts in this world. For there in Atlanta, my hemophilia, the one thing that I had thought would define my life from birth to death, had been utterly, totally, and permanently cured.

Time AND *Space*

*The future is an infinite succession of presents, and
to live now as we think human beings should live,
in defiance of all that is bad around us, is itself a
marvelous victory.*

—HOWARD ZINN

I am once again sitting in Maine in the small log cabin to which I have been returning for more than fifty years. The sun is rising through the fir trees and warming the tall grass. A breeze is blowing straight up from the cove, carrying the rich aroma of ocean and sand, seaweed and clay, all brushed clean by the forest. Bees are making their rounds of the black-eyed Susans and blue cornflowers planted just in front of my window, while an emerald-backed hummingbird flutters from blossom to blossom. It is now more than two years since my transplant and my startling return to activity.

As I sit, I wonder, what does one do with a second chance in life?

Under any normal circumstance, I should not be here. When I was born, hemophilia was considered a potentially fatal illness; my life expectancy was less than thirty years. When I contracted HIV, the usual amount of time between diagnosis, progression to AIDS, and death was as little as two years and no more than five. And each year thousands of people in the United States—and millions around the world—die of liver disease from hepatitis C.

Yet here I am, sitting quietly and at peace, my hemophilia resolved, my HIV tamed by my immune system and medication, and my hepatitis rolled back through the advent of a new liver. In my fifties, I am still alive—and I am now at liberty to die of old age.

*

Sidelined and silenced for long periods of time, I am now healed and feeling new force. I am no longer a racehorse trapped in a barn; the doors have been unlocked, the gates have been thrown open, and I can see the rolling fields of the future sparkling in the sun and stretching to the horizon. I now want to go out into the world and to speak and to act, not for myself but for everyone who is struggling and hoping for a better life. I see a great deal of what is wrong with our economy and our world, and I want to join those who are seeking to renew democracy and to transform our economy into one that is newly prosperous and sustainable.

In short, I have a simple yet immense desire. I want everyone to thrive. Each person and each family deserves the right to enjoy the relatively brief time we have been allotted on this planet. To do so, they need access to the basic foundations of a life of dignity and prosperity. In America many of our old solutions and institutions have failed, and it is time for us to take bold steps to create new ones.

I want to work so that every family has the basics of life: a good home, a good school, a good doctor, and a good job. These four walls together form a foundation of freedom and prosperity. When we look around the country, we see too many people struggling to obtain these basics. There are many reasons for such struggles, from personal problems to market failures to structural injustice. But a life, a community, and a nation that provides these things is not some magical fantasy. It was the purpose of the founders and has been the goal of every subsequent generation. The question that burns within me now is whether this is still our goal today. Or have we, for the first time in American history, lost confidence in our dreams?

My conviction is clear. After having lived through all the events detailed in this book, I believe that our direction is determined by the blend of our aspirations and our desires. It *matters* what we choose to believe in.

If I had listened to the conventional wisdom about my health, I would have resigned myself to an early death and never set foot outside the apparently small, sad domain of my life. If millions of people had listened to what was said about racism in the United States and South Africa, then we would not have worked tirelessly for racial equality. Nelson Mandela would have died in prison, and the people he brought together would have remained trapped in the division, misery, and hatred that seemed at one point to be their only destiny. There never would have been an African-American president of the United States. If we had given up on the ideal that we must preserve our planet, we would never have created the institutions and practices that are setting us on a common path toward sustainable prosperity.

Our values guide our choices before we act. We design blueprints before we build. As it says in the New Testament, hope is faith in things *not* seen. Every course is set by pointing to a destination where we have yet to arrive.

As a nation we have faced deeply discouraging moments before. Our union almost dissolved many times in its first hundred years. And even though we may not break into two physical nations, we are no longer "one nation, indivisible, with liberty and justice for all." The United States has become a nation divided by dollars. Many Americans are still reeling under the hammer blows of wild market forces and financial manipulation. The poor and the wealthy now live in such isolation from each other that they often forget they are citizens of the same country.

We have been resilient because of our inner strength and our dynamic institutions. American achievements are so large and so astonishing that we actually forget to speak about them and thus learn their lessons. Consider what we have already done. In a few decades at the beginning of the nation, we established bustling ports and built factories that competed with the greatest empires of the day. We tied two oceans together through a web of railroad tracks and canals. We created thousands of extraordinary inventions, everything from the flat broom to the light bulb, from electric current to refrigeration, from the telephone to television. All came from a single country that did not have a population over 100 million until the 1920s. We invented the automobile and the airplane. Then came radar and radio, the transistor, the atomic bomb, the microchip, the computer, and the Internet. We walked on the moon. Earlier generations would have seen the abilities that we now take for granted as the powers of gods.

How can anyone, faced with the most radical transformation in technology in the history of human civilization, argue that the world is not primarily driven by ideas? Who can say that something to which we might aspire today is automatically impossible? They cannot. The question is not *can* we do something, but what do we *want* to do?

I often think about how much the nation we call "the United States" has evolved within a few generations of one family. My great-grandfather Robert Kinloch Massie was born in 1864 into a Virginia family of modest farmers and middle-level gentry whose livelihood depended on land they had already held for nearly two hundred years, most of which was worked by slaves. They were Christians and Americans, and they believed in the brotherhood of man and the ideals of the United States, yet their economic interest and cultural training blinded them from extending these principles to the women and the slaves in their midst. They were living a terrible contradiction, though to them it was not obvious—and indeed, the thought may never have occurred to them at all.

Their lives were thrown into moral, political, and economic chaos during the Civil War. They watched their sons and cousins die on the battlefields, they abandoned their belief in slavery, they sold or lost their farms, and they moved into town to pursue various learned professions. My great-grandfather eventually became a minister and left the United States to become a missionary and schoolteacher in China. His son, my grandfather, was born far from the American South, in Shanghai, in 1891. The family eventually returned and settled in the United States again, first in Virginia and then permanently in Kentucky, which is where my father appeared, in 1929. During much of this same period the members of my mother's family were going about their lives in the towns and mountain villages of Switzerland, with no thought that some of them would ever move to the new English-speaking empire rising thousands of miles away. Every person comes from such a succession of families filled with such twists and turns in their history.

Consider the political changes that we eventually achieved in our country through argument and agreement. We implemented the principle of free and compulsory education for all children. We set aside millions of acres and billions of dollars for public schools and universities. We fought an agonizing civil war, full of waste, denial, brutality, and suffering, but it achieved the goal of ending slavery. The nation delayed its political promise to women for an unacceptable amount of time, but after a protracted struggle, America embraced women's suffrage. We fought tyranny in two world wars. After long and shameful denial, we finally faced up to the obvious conclusions of our own principles and ended segregation. We installed a first line of defense against the poisoning of our water and air. And now, after asking Americans to look deeply into their hearts about the nature of love, we are moving toward the universal acceptance of gay marriage.

None of this was easy. It all required vision, courage, and leadership. And it all happened, in historical terms, in the twinkling of an eye. Who says the eye cannot twinkle again?

Together we now must create a new, more fair, more prosperous, and more just America. To do so, we must measure and manage the things that matter to us as a whole people. Economic growth is one piece of the puzzle. A new American economy would enable us to chart our course so that our communities are improving, our children are learning, our workers are finding meaningful work, our natural world is flourishing, our cities are becoming safer and more beautiful.

All of this comes back to the concept of sustainability, which governs discussion throughout the world but is still barely mentioned in the United States. Sustainability is a point of dynamic equilibrium where all the forces for good—our creative gifts, our economic genius, our skillful use of resources, our desire for freedom and happiness, our longing for comfort and convenience, our reverence for the dignity of every human life—come together. It recognizes the diversity of goals among the seven billion people who live on the planet and balances them effectively with all the other biological forces at work in the world to create a system that not only works for us but will last for generations.

Sustainability is an improved and logical progression within capitalism. It expands the definition of capitalism to acknowledge what we already know: that there are different forms of capital, such as financial capital, natural capital, human capital, and intellectual capital. The goal of an economy should not be to deplete one form of capital in favor of another—for example, mowing down life-giving rain forests or stripping the vitality of workers in order to obtain short-term financial returns—but to create systems that allow every capital stock to increase.

The good news is that this is already happening. The conversations and actions are already taking place in hundreds of groups and communities around the United States. One can find new names for new ideas and thus bring them into sight. And powerful institutions are moving to put the pieces in place. To give one example, the largest accounting societies and firms in the world are now working with the Global Reporting Initiative, under the overall sponsorship of the Prince of Wales and the United Nations, to merge sustainability and financial accounting into a single tool for measuring corporate performance. If they succeed, the way corporations are financed, rewarded, managed, and structured will be transformed.

An effort to change the entire world economy might seem like folly, an enterprise too large to imagine, let alone to achieve. Yet if one can imagine a different world, that new world already starts to shimmer into view. Most human practice is the result of social convention. We have learned from America's struggles with race, gender, disability, and sexual orientation, that as ideas about social convention change, so do practices and laws.

Consider how far we could go if we regarded our current challenges through the very simple lenses of innovation and investment. Innovation and investment both focus on the future. They involve the creation or exchange of something today in order to generate a larger benefit tomorrow. They testify that everything is interrelated.

In the field of energy, we know that innovation means moving away from our excessive reliance on fossil fuel by expanding renewable energy, improving efficiency, and creating new energy sources. These are the right things to do economically and the right things to do morally and scientifically, given the large-scale climate crisis bearing down on the planet.

In education we also have tremendous opportunities. The nineteenth-century model of pouring children into a classroom for part of the day to listen to one adult is not a complete model. Through the Internet it will be possible within our lifetimes to provide education for everyone everywhere for free.

We can go through every major problem facing America and show how a commitment to innovation and investment would chart a course for progress. In foreign and military policy, we need to create new networks and relationships with other countries so that we strengthen the web of interconnections and the power of American ideals within the global system. In medicine, we are constantly innovating, but we are not making the results—from which I have personally benefited—evenly available. And in dealing with our democracy, we must continue to create new ways to bring our citizens—particularly our young people—more into the political process. As we do so, we must put an end to the tsunami of secret money flooding into our elections to corrupt our elected officials.

The creation of a sustainable economy built on innovation and investment, leading to justice and prosperity, is a large goal, but no more challenging, and no less worthy than many that the United States has already achieved.

*

To make these changes, we are going to need to let go of some of the labels we employ to classify each other. They harm our judgment and taint our souls. And we are always bigger and deeper than the names others apply to us.

For my whole life I have been a Christian, because on balance I have believed that this term captures my belief in God and many other strong and worthy ideas about how people should be guided in their decisions and relations to each other. Yet I recognize that some people who call themselves Christians have done hateful things that I reject, and that I bear the risk of being tarnished by that name because of the poor judgment and bad behavior of others.

I have devoted thousands of hours to leadership as an environmentalist, yet I would dearly like to find another name for that movement, since it seems to me that anything with the term *mentalist* in it automatically sounds somewhat loopy.

Though I have long been a Democrat, I understand the passion of the members of the Tea Party to discover and bring to the surface the original motivations of our revolutionary founders, though having made my own study of these leaders, I believe that many are drawing the wrong conclusions. The authors of the American Revolution never believed in moving backward in time, as the Tea Party seems to insist on doing— they believed in balancing political stability and invention, sometimes in enormously creative and risky ways. The true legacy of the American Revolution is that we must continue to refine and improve our democracy until a more perfect union, a government of the people, by the people, and for the people, has been fully achieved.

Let us choose a new way of talking to each other that honors each other's dignity even as we disagree, perhaps profoundly, with each other's views. Even though I have fought passionately for the ideas that I believe are right for this country and this world, I want everyone to be reminded of the mysterious nobility of life itself. We need terms that offer dignity, honor, and respect to our souls.

We need a term for those who are profoundly in love with the privilege of being alive.

We need a term for those who stand in awe of the beauty of the whole world—from gardeners and hunters and astronauts to nurses, from mountain climbers and sunbathers and skiers to pilots, from explorers and fishermen to farmers, from scientists and painters and poets to dancers, from old people breathing their last breath to children putting their first toe into the water.

We need a term for anyone who straightens up from a tractor, glances out the window of an office, strolls through a park, hikes through a forest, or turns a face upward to meet a summer rain and feel a moment of release.

We need a term for those who desire to work without causing harm, and to eat and to drink with gratitude, for those who long to sing and to laugh and to see the sun rise again to signal the dawn of a new day.

We need a term for the huge majority of us who want to use our time and talents to create new chances for beauty, who want to dwell in peace and reverence for the gifts that have been given to us for millions of years for free.

And, truthfully, we already know what that term is.

It is *human being*.

What does one do with a second chance in life? That is a question not only for me but for every person, and for our world as a whole.

Personally, I am going to take on the struggle, with all my passion and with all my flaws, and with as many allies as I can assemble, to find the path to prosperity and sustainability, from whatever side, and in whatever place, so that humans may be seen for what they often are and what they always can become: honorable, strong, responsible, and beautiful. Others have given to me, and within whatever time is still mine I want to give back.

I want to share the secret that was lying in plain sight for my whole life but that only became clear to me when I awoke from my brush with eternity. And that truth is that every person and every community, as a function of our free will, can always find a second chance. Every instant offers the gift of renewal. The choice for each of us and all of us is whether we choose to see and embrace that moment.

The world may have its structures and consequences, but it is also full of grace that confers healing and freedom. That is the blessing of our residence on this lovely planet, which, no matter what we dream or do, will continue to spin gently into the future across an infinite ocean of stars.

Acknowledgments

Most of what I have been able to do in life has been the result of the generosity and assistance of others, so it is daunting to try to thank people in a short statement. To everyone mentioned in the book, and the many more friends and family members who are not, I offer my gratitude for your many years of love and support. Your compassion and affection have made my life not only possible but wonderful.

I owe a special thanks to those who helped bring this book into being and who assisted us during the difficult years described in the last part.

Over the years people have encouraged me to write a memoir as a sequel to my parents' book *Journey*. In that book, first published in 1975 and reissued with a new epilogue in 1984, my parents described my childhood with hemophilia. I started on a much longer autobiographical work during the years I was ill, but then I realized that my life might outrun my pages and that I should speed up the process.

In 2011 I had the opportunity to deliver a Grand Rounds

lecture at Brigham and Women's Hospital in Boston, and I concentrated on telling five particular anecdotes from different moments in my life. The reaction proved so strong and positive that I decided to expand those stories into this memoir. I also spent much of 2011 as a candidate for the United States Senate in Massachusetts, and I wanted to offer the public an accounting of the origins and nature of my thinking. Though the campaign came to a premature close in late 2011 because of changing political circumstances, it was a wonderful experience. I thank the members of my campaign team, including Ali Denosky-Smart, Eleanor Fort, Dave Kartunen, Sam Levor, Pat Tomaino, Lynda Wik, and Matt Wilson, as well as my great interns and volunteers. They all worked hard to move the campaign forward every day, even as their candidate set aside the early morning hours to write. I salute you and thank you for believing in the democratic process.

I had many conversations at key moments that infused me with the necessary spirit to tackle this project. Chuck Collins got me fired up over lunch. Allen White offered his usual wise counsel even as he was meeting new challenges of his own. I want to single out the exceptional contribution of Owen Andrews, who met with me frequently to talk about themes; sifted through old speeches, diaries, and articles to find stories; and offered excellent editorial counsel throughout the process. With his help, I was able to focus the chapters and get them written much more swiftly than would otherwise have been possible.

The enthusiasm and professional wisdom offered by Melanie Jackson, my friend and literary agent, proved invaluable. I am deeply honored to have had the chance to work again with my editor and publisher, Nan A. Talese, who not only believed in the idea of the book but repeatedly added her elegant handwriting to the manuscript with an unerring eye as to how to make it better. With insight, diplomacy, and skill, she coaxes the very best from all of her writers, and I am fortunate to be one of them.

I want to offer special appreciation to some of the physicians who are not mentioned or are mentioned only briefly in this book, but to whom I turned for many years for assistance, including Dennis Burke, Stephen Chanock, Raymond Chung, Kathleen Corey, Winston Hewitt, Christopher Hughes, Stuart Knechtle, James Markmann, Sameer Mazhar, Sandra Nelson, Eric Rosenberg, R. Malcolm Smith, Owen Surmann, and Bruce Walker. They offered their professional skill and their personal friendship without hesitation or limit. I also thank Jean Pearce Handler and her lovely family, without whom this story would have turned out very differently.

I owe a special debt to the additional doctors, physical therapists, technicians, and especially the extraordinary nurses who gave generously of their time and talent to help me survive, endure, and recover after many medical challenges. I know I speak for everyone they have touched, standing rank upon rank to the horizon, when I say thank you.

A large circle of family and friends gathered around us over the past ten years to lift us up and move us forward.

Our neighbor Ed Lavelle, who can fix anything, took care of many necessary repairs to our old house. My sister Elizabeth stepped in to gather information and rally support at a moment when we had nearly lost hope. All the other members of Anne's family and mine made unique and important contributions. The members of St. James's Episcopal Church in Cambridge, Massachusetts, cared for us over many years, offering us meals, prayers, friendship, and innumerable acts of gentle support. My sons, Sam and John, provided vital help and affection even as they set out on their excellent new paths in life. During the past few years, when I was struggling and recovering from illness, my daughter, Kate, showed strength, patience, and compassion far beyond her years, and she has blossomed into an extraordinary young woman. Katie, the dedication of this book will show you that I listen to you (and love you) more than you will ever know.

The person who cared the most, bore the most, worried the most, and loved the most has been my wife, Anne. She was present through all the hidden suffering and joy. A beacon of hope at all moments, she guided me through and brought me home.

The arcing years align in sight
to bathe us both in blessing light;
They help us see beneath the smile;
beneath the mind, the will, the guile;
Beneath the swirl of gives and takes;

beneath the grief, missteps, mistakes
To find ourselves by grace subdued
returned, restored, reborn, renewed.
And so to you, my dearly wife,
I deed my longing, love, and life.

A NOTE ABOUT THE AUTHOR

BOB MASSIE is an American environmental leader, author, Episcopal priest, and former anti-apartheid activist. He created or led three of the world's leading sustainability organizations: Ceres, the Global Reporting Initiative, and the Investor Network on Climate Risk. His book *Loosing the Bonds: The United States and South Africa in the Apartheid Years* won the Lionel Gelber Prize for the best book on international relations in 1998.

Pierre Simon Fournier *le jeune,* who designed the type used in this book, was both an originator and a collector of types. His services to the art of printing were his design of letters, his creation of ornaments and initials, and his standardization of type sizes. His types are old style in character and sharply cut. In 1764 and 1766 he published his *Manuel typographique,* a treatise on the history of French types and printing, on typefounding in all its details, and on what many consider his most important contribution to typography—the measurement of type by the point system.